The Life of Brian

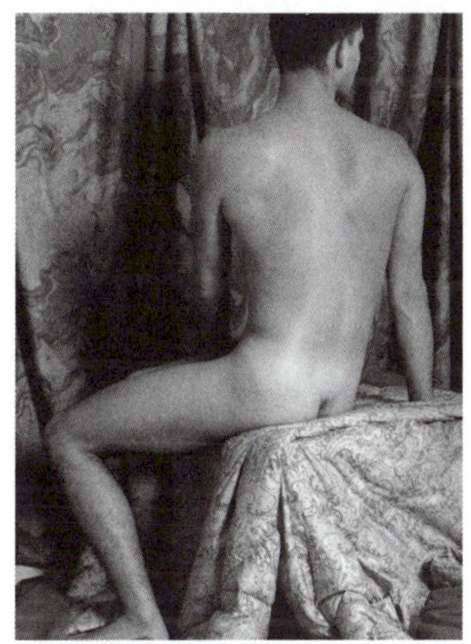

The Life of Brian

Masculinities, Sexualities and Health in New Zealand

EDITED BY
HEATHER WORTH, ANNA PARIS
AND LOUISA ALLEN

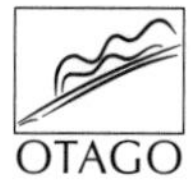

OTAGO

University of Otago Press
PO Box 56/56 Union Street West
Dunedin, New Zealand
Fax: 64 3 479 8385
Email: university.press@otago.a.c.nz

First published 2002

ISBN 1 877276 25 1

Cover image: *The Heart's Vision*, 1988, by Fiona Pardington.
Gelatin silver print gold-toned. 38 x 28 cm.
Printed in New Zealand by Astra Print Ltd, Wellington

Contents

Preface

This collection of essays grew from a 'Masculinities' conference, organised by Heather Worth, Alison Jones and Anna Paris in July 2000 at the University of Auckland. Despite theatrical weather, a group of interested people from within the academic and wider community, national and international, came together to share ideas and recent developments in both theorising and working within the area of masculinities. What emerged from this conference was a strong emphasis on issues of health and sexualities within the wider context of theorising masculinities. The conference also elicited a call for more research into masculinities within Aotearoa/New Zealand. This collection of essays is our contribution to what is emerging as a fascinating and timely study of contemporary masculinities, sexualities and health.

How is it that three women are editing a volume on masculinity and male health and sexuality? All three of us have an interest in the area. Heather Worth's work, particularly, has focused on gay men's sexuality and HIV. Louisa Allen's doctoral research examined both young men's and young women's experiences of sex and heterosexuality. We don't, however, want to claim any special expertise, and we do see our role in this collection as conduits for those working in what is an under-represented area. Surveying the field prior to writing this introduction, we have been shocked at just how little work is being done and we would encourage New Zealand scholars to take up the challenge and get to work 'out there'.

We would like to acknowledge the hard work of all the contributors to the book, the support of the Institute for Research on Gender board of management for their encouragement to publish, and above all Associate Professor Alison Jones for her trust in us.

HEATHER WORTH, ANNA PARIS AND LOUISA ALLEN

Preface

TO JONATHAN, SIMON AND ANDREW

Introduction

Anna Paris, Heather Worth and Louisa Allen

> He's not the Son of God. He's just a naughty boy!
> (Monty Python's *Life of Brian*)

It has only been in the last few decades that an academic interest in the study of masculinities has been seen as important, even necessary, to a more complete understanding of the ways class, culture, society, race and sexuality intersect to produce bodies of a particularly masculine configuration. In fact, a quick look through the available literature on this topic reveals a thin veil of academic interest in theorising the subject. Despite Connell's (1995: iv) claim that 'there has been an impressive growth of social science research on masculinity'[1] over the last decade, we would argue that this is largely indebted to the advances in feminist theory, with its broadening into areas such as gender and, theoretically inevitably, perhaps, the study of masculinities.

Defining masculinities

The study of 'masculinities' cannot proceed without properly defining what the term actually refers to, and how, in a number of ways, we might begin to find answers. R.W. Connell, in his book *Masculinities*, well referenced in this publication, distinguishes and identifies essentialist definitions, positivist social science, normative definitions, and semiotic approaches to the study of masculinities.[2] He describes 'masculinity' as:

> ... simultaneously a place in gender relations, the practices through which men and women engage that place in gender, and the effects of these practices in bodily experience, personality and culture.[3]

George L. Mosse is more broad and simplistic in his approach, defining masculinity as 'the way men assert what they believe to be their manhood'.[4] In any case, masculinities is more than the idea of the macho, or hyper-masculine: most often it is considered to be the socially constructed gender attributed to the male sex. Like the notion of the 'feminine', it is saturated with attributed and associated meaning. It is this 'meaning' that we seek to extract from the discursively complex and sometimes contradictory masculine subject. Thus the study of masculinities contests long-held notions of 'inherent masculinity': the lack of academic inquiry into the study of 'the masculine' is a result of a history of regarding the experiences and behaviours of the male gender as fixed and static, and as a benchmark from which to measure feminine modes of behaviour.

Approaches to studying masculinity – the sex/gender argument

> Gender terms are contested because the right to account for gender is claimed by conflicting discourses and systems of knowledge.[5]

Three areas of study have dominated the study of masculinity during the course of the twentieth century. Clinical knowledge, based on and stemming from Freudian theory, remains the first attempt to create and develop a science of masculinity. Jungian theory and the development of psychoanalysis followed in its wake. Social psychology utilised the 'normative sex -role' theory in order to frame and understand the masculine subject, and this became part of mainstream-speak in the social sciences of the 1950s. However, recent developments in anthropology, history and sociology have contested the sex-role theory, acknowledging the multitudes of variations possible in attempting to create an understanding of masculinities.

The notion of 'masculinity' is not universal. The embodiment of masculinity is specific to the culture and historical moment to which it belongs. Experiences of masculinity are intersected and defined by class, ethnicity, race and sexualities, and are as diverse as such intersections will allow. Further, the concept of masculinity does not exist except in relation and contrast to 'femininity'. This is to say: there is nothing inherent to masculinity, all is defined in contrast to what it is understood to be *not.*

In light of this, a rethinking of masculinities may begin by acknowledging that, in our culture at least, 'the physical sense of maleness and femaleness is central to the cultural interpretation of gender'.[6] So the very corporeal experience of embodying masculinity, of embracing corporeality, is a basis from which we may theorise masculinities.

The conception of 'what it is to be a man' is culturally, historically and socially specific. The specific nature of masculinity, even in New Zealand, means that we cannot speak or assume that there is a universal experience of the masculine. As Phillips argues, 'the character of the Pakeha male stereotype in New Zealand was forged by ... the desire to keep alive the muscular virtues of the pioneer heritage, and the concern to contain that masculine spirit within respectable boundaries'.[7] So the image of Brian (Brian Lohore, perhaps?), the much-loved 'kiwi bloke' is really a construction of ideals, specific to a certain geographics/demographics and time in modern history, rather than a biologically inevitable result of being a man in New Zealand. And this idealisation, as Judith Butler has argued (1993), is impossible to realise. This masculinity (and its other, femininity) is a site of ambivalence, lack or loss.

RETHINKING THE CORPOREAL AS PREREQUISITE FOR THE STUDY OF MASCULINITY

The academic study of the male gender, like that of the female (via feminist and women's studies), is not simple or well defined. On the one hand, the study of masculinities involves acknowledging the notion of gender as floating, as not intrinsically anchored to the sexed body.[8] It also involves a realisation that what makes up the masculine gender is a continuum of behaviours, expectations, experiences, institutions, structures, systems and ideas about what it means 'to be a man'.

The study of masculinities involves a re-negotiation of the body within sociological discourse. In order to undertake such a study, we need to think about what it is we are actually examining, and what our assumptions and bases for discussion will be. The major debate within the social sciences during the twentieth century has been the premise from those of the socio-biological persuasion that gender is a result of belonging to a particular body, which carries with it genetic material, historical predispositions and hormonal patterns. The sexed body – in this case, the male body – is the major determinant of much behaviour, actions and experiences. In opposition to this perspective is the sociological argument, which places primary importance on processes of socialisation, institutions, and systems, as well as cultural, historical and gendered expectations. These result in the body becoming gendered to a particular configuration of the ideal. The socio-biological argument depends upon the body as chemical, as blood, bone and neuro-functioning; the sociological views the body as a discursively conceived surface upon which inscriptions of normative masculinity are inscribed, to varying degrees of permanence. However, Butler argues that:

> if gender is the cultural meanings that the sexed body assumes, then a gender cannot be said to follow from a sex in any one way ... it does not follow that the construction of 'men' will accrue exclusively to the bodies of males or that 'women' will interpret only female bodies ...When the constructed status of gender is theorised as radically independent of sex, gender itself becomes a free-floating artifice, with the consequence that man and masculine might just as easily signify a female body as a male one, and woman and feminine a male body as easily as a female one.[9]

Re-thinking materiality in this way allows for more radical configurations of the masculine, as posed in this book. To a large extent, however, the subject of inquiry, the subject of the masculine, might well be considered as being at a flux in time, whereby an open and fluid definition of the subject is content for a moment, to remain a site of contested knowledges and interpretations. Hence we talk about 'masculinities' rather than the singular 'masculinity'. This is in acknowledgement of the diverse and many ways in which masculinity can be interpreted, 'worn', acted out and embodied, and this plurality seeks to be inclusive of all experiences of 'being a man'. It is also a way by which we can bypass the problem of 'speaking for all men' – that is, of assuming that the experiences of masculinity are shared by all men. Acknowledging the multitudes of possible masculinities is an important step forward to a more inclusive and thorough development of a study of masculinities.

Why study New Zealand masculinities?

Why study New Zealand masculinities and what will we do with this knowledge? Notions of masculinity in this country impact on every area of public and private life, from the complex power relations in the family sphere to the phallic attributes of the advanced consumer capitalist politics of the New Right. Further, the quest to embody the 'kiwi bloke' – the strong, silent type who enjoys a few beers with his mates, watches rugby, and likes a bet on the horses every now and then – has had definite consequences for men in terms of poor levels of health, and high rates of imprisonment, domestic violence, suicide and divorce.

Undercutting the grim statistics measuring these social problems is a reluctance to let go of an unrealistic, out-of-date but nostalgic ideal of masculinity that is peculiar to New Zealand, with its history of pioneering, biculturalism and rugby. With the challenges of second-wave feminism in the 1960s, 70s and 80s, the gay movement of the 1980s leading to an increasingly legitimated 'out' gay culture, and an increasingly disapproving public discourse on domestic violence, the notion of 'what it means to be a man' is changing.

The purpose of this book is therefore to examine some of the ways in which the contemporary embodiment of masculinity is experienced, and how it has changed from previous generations that saw deviation from the narrowly defined idea of the kiwi bloke as largely repugnant. Secondly, the book will explore the diversity encompassed within the 'new' masculine experience, with its contradictions, its differences, and its hopes for the future. The acknowledgement of diversity is essential to a more complete understanding of what masculinity means.

Jock Phillips' *A Man's Country* remains a watershed in terms of a New Zealand work recognising the Pakeha kiwi male as worthy of academic study. 'Barry Crump' look-alikes, featuring inborn skills with fencing wire and construction work, were what made New Zealand men special, unique, charming.

Traditionally associated with notions of strength, potency, knowledge, leadership and (hetero)sexual prowess, the 'average' New Zealand male may not match up to these lofty ideals. It has been only in recent times that the inquiry into masculinities has sought to recognise and take seriously a wider range of possibility for men. The acceptance of diversity within the male gender has become necessary for understanding how New Zealand men today experience their lives and their relationships, their bodies and their gender. Times are changing.

SEXUALITY

How can we think Brian's sexuality? Little has been written about male heterosexuality: the writing on male sexuality in New Zealand which has begun to appear has almost singularly concentrated on homosexuality.[10] It seems almost impossible to unpack the 'taken-for-granted' dominant heterosexuality found here, as it appears to exist only as the other's 'other'. In other words, we examine kiwi heterosexuality only in opposition to either female sexuality or to homosexuality.

Some scholarly attention elsewhere has been paid to psychoanalytic theories of male sexuality,[11] and an attendant emphasis on the unconscious and its importance in the constitution of male subjectivity. However, social constructionist approaches, which view male sexuality as something historically and culturally constituted through relations of power, have been the major theoretical tools of those studying male sexuality in the last two decades.[12] Here, we view male sexuality as a discursive-technological complex which attaches itself to bodies and pleasures.[13] We argue that sexuality and the sexed subject are not transcendental signifiers with universal referents, neither are they underlying biological essences with drives and instincts, but concepts that came into being at a certain historical period. Sex is a conglomeration of elements – physiological processes, muscular activities, wishes, hopes, desires, sensations, attitudes, knowledge, while sexuality is nothing other than an artificial constructed unity or effect of a relationship between power, knowledge and bodily pleasure.

How, then, did Brian get to be the sexual subject he is today, what technologies of the body and discourses of truth have constituted and managed his sexuality? This introduction can only approach the subject, for the history of New Zealand sexuality has yet to be written. But we can say that, in the case of kiwi men, sexuality (as the site of (re)productivity) has been forged through the nineteenth-century imperialist necessity for land, life and labour. New Zealand male (Pakeha) virility has been drawn from the harsh conditions in which Pakeha men found themselves on arrival here. For Maori men, of course, little is known about pre-colonisation gender, sexuality and masculinity.

One might argue that a new kind of (hetero)sexual identity was formed in New Zealand (and in other parts of the new world), an identity very much based on the physical body, on movement from place to place, on solitude and mateship. According to Foucault,[14] bodies are necessary to the productivity of modernity for they are wholly present, strong forces. Hard physical labour characterised the early colonial era, and the movement of whalers, sealers, labourers, goldminers, gumdiggers, shearers and swaggers around the country meant men's sexuality was largely unfettered. Men often spent long periods alone and solitude has been a recurring theme in New Zealand fiction, but at the same time as Phillips argues, 'frontier conditions often forced [men] into a close comradeship .... [However,] the character of this mateship should not be misconstrued. It was rarely a passionate or enduring friendship between two men'.[15]

A particularly kiwi style or technique of male sexuality was forged in these colonial conditions, a style which prevails as a dominant ideal. Under frontier conditions, the sex trade burgeoned. Eldred-Grigg shows that in Christchurch 23 brothels and 80 full-time sex workers were known to the police by 1859, and by 1864 200 prostitutes were resident in Dunedin.[16] This anarchy of bodies and pleasures was not to last. In the second half of the nineteenth century the tension between public sexuality and the desire to civilise the wilderness began to manifest itself. The bourgeois family needed to take its rightful place in the new world. Not only had Edward Gibbon Wakefield envisaged colonisation by families and the transplantation of old-world hierarchies and social order, but there was a growing middle class in the cities and small towns.[17] Marriage and the family were seen as the answer to the drifting single man and his unregulated sexuality.

Alongside the growing imperative for a new kind of New Zealand family man with a managed and regulated sexuality came prohibitionary moves on alcohol and prostitution. Legislation – such as the Contagious Diseases Act (1869) against the spread of venereal disease, the Criminal Code of 1893 which made brothel-keeping punishable by imprisonment, and the Police Offences Amendment Act of 1901 which criminalised pimping – was introduced and passed into law. But as Phillips argues, 'the chief remedy for male sexual vice in the opinion of the respectable was a moral code of self-control. Men had to learn to curb their appetites'.[18]

The First World War interrupted these regulating moves over the bodies of New Zealand men. While the war was central in the development of both nationhood and masculinity, as well as the preservation of imperial virility, soldiers used the war as a way of loosening the hold of the encroaching domestic sphere. For instance, Ettie Rout, the pioneering family-planner, saw men's chastity in war as 'quite impractical'.[19] Casual sexuality abounded, with a concomitant high incidence of VD, although few men made mention of it in their diaries or letters home.[20] But at the end of the war, there were renewed efforts to bring men back into line. Male sexuality again became a means of, and was burdened by, social control, regulated through increasing demands for labour and reproduction, and inserted 'into the machinery of [re]production'.[21] Sex became an individual, private, nuclear family matter. The reaction to this enforced domesticity was not positive. As Phillips argues, a man had 'a special need to keep the domestic responsibilities at a distance, lest in becoming a family man he was stripped of his virile identity'.[22] Male sexuality, then, was a site of a continual tension between the public and the private.

However, the management of kiwi male sexuality occurred not by repression, but through a network of norms that induced a certain kind of sexuality. For example, in 1922 a committee of the Board of Health was appointed to investigate venereal disease. The recommendation of the committee placed the burden on education. Self-control was the answer to male sexual excess: 'Self-reverence, self-knowledge, self-control – these three alone lead life to sovereign power'.[23] Through its prohibition, sex became the most important part of men's and boy's lives, a positivity that has transformed and managed sexuality. Disciplinary statements such as the above constituted the sexual normalisation of the New Zealand male through a network of institutions, discourses, education and, above all, through self-knowledge and self-surveillance. This elaboration of discourses of sexuality developed at the same time as sex became the focus of continual public debate. As Foucault argues:

> the manifold mechanisms which, in the areas of economy, pedagogy, medicine, and justice, incite, extract, distribute, and institutionalise the sexual discourse, an immense verbosity is what our civilisation has required and organised.[24]

The context underlying the discourses of sexuality are not only the social, the political, and the economic but also the raw material of the body. The body and its practices are the privileged and productive targets of power, and sexuality the *dispositif par excellence* around which the body is disciplined and trained. In New Zealand, from the early part of the twentieth century, rugby was seen as a particular technique of body management. Rugby was considered to be a way of obtaining self-control, and also a physical release. A report on an investigation into the Burnham Industrial School in 1906 recommended, as an antidote to the boys' sexual degeneracy, sport (and in particular, rugby): rugby would act as a sexual sublimation.[25] Truby King also encouraged sport as a way for boys 'to maintain supremacy over themselves and those innate tendencies which have to be fought with and mastered'.[26] The 'problematic of the flesh' could be solved through positive and healthy pleasures.

But, rugby not only privileges bodies, it also eroticises them. The disciplining of the body through rugby realigned bodily pleasure and also intensified it.

Rugby has become intimately connected to male sexual functioning. Lynne Star argues that 'elite rugby players are possessed of a mythical elusive and potent sexuality symbolised in the game itself'.[27] And as she and Nick Perry have claimed, its overarching televisualisation has meant that rugby has become a primal scene of homosociality and even homoeroticism:

> Then everything seems to go into slow motion like some kind of replay on the TV. I see myself running across the field and I see Joe pass the ball to Errol, and Errol to Willy and I'm dodging in and out and the crowd's shouting, and Willy passes to me and I'm just about over the line and somebody tackles me. And it's Stick. And he's on top of me. And he's right up inside me, fucking me.[28]

Rugby players are objects of male desire. Yet central to the kiwi psyche was the claim that rugby was 'emphatically not a game for poofters'.[29] And it is true that rugby's wrapping of 'the sexual body in its embrace',[30] is not solely homoerotic. Watching rugby is certainly pleasurable for women,[31] and a sign of heterosexual virility. As Michael King writes:

> Perhaps we associated sex with sport because our adolescent rugby careers unfolded at the same time as sexuality. And although this was never made clear to us at the time, one of the reasons for placing so much emphasis on sport was to sublimate sexual impulses. An idle mind was the devil's workshop and so was an idle body. Paradoxically, although it may have reduced the incidence of self-abuse, the machismo swagger that seemed part of being superbly fit also nudged us towards exaggerated feelings of sexual competence and fantasies about how we could conquer women.[32]

Rugby players could score on and off the field.

The apparatus of sexuality, as a heterogeneous body of laws, institutions and statements about sex, has made sexuality central to the development of the kiwi male subject. Brian's sexuality has become the deepest truth of his self or subjectivity. Brian has become a subject of desire.[33] Kevin Ireland says of his adolescence:

> We bumbled along in pursuit of some desperate notion we had of sex, composed of furtive guesswork in the appropriately named pillbox, the misinformation of yarns and smutty jokes, confusions from sex manuals and encyclopaedias, rows of dots in steamy books and misunderstandings of all kinds, fuelled by a physical appetite.[34]

And as Michael King says, 'sex, raw sex was a source of insatiable interest'.[35] Jock Phillips discovered his sexuality at about the age of fourteen when a chemistry experiment:

> Started a practice of competitive sexual discovery among my mates that was an education in itself. At first, although we fantasised endlessly about girls, masturbation remained the centre of discussion. We would arrive in the morning and compare notes about speed and quantity. The real thing came closer, when dancing lessons began .... The only thing of interest to your mates on Monday was not 'How did you get on?', but 'How far did you get?'. We would spend the

> lunchtimes in competitive comparisons of 'how far' we had been allowed 'to get'.[36]

What is peculiar about New Zealand society, is the dedication with which young men dedicated themselves to speaking of sex *ad infinitum.*[37] Sexuality is not purely an object of familial or institutional scrutiny; as boys feel their sexuality is under observation they begin to exercise a sexual surveillance over themselves, which lasts their lifetime. Sam Hunt had this to say about his Catholic boyhood:

> My first confession was with Father Kelly. I said, 'Bless me Father for I have sinned, this is my First Confession' and so on.
> 'And what do have to confess, child?' from behind the grille.
> 'I've been impure in my actions.'
> 'What do you mean? Touching yourself?'
> 'Yes.'
> 'Where?'
> 'Where else?'
> 'How many times?'
> A seven-year-old kid! All I could think of was that there were 365 days in a year so I took a stab at it and said, 'Three hundred and sixty-five.'
> I suppose I got three Hail Marys and went away rejoicing.[38]

Self-knowledge has become integral to desire. Through self-examination sexuality can be knowable, and any deviation from the norm able to be exposed and dealt with. In this sense kiwi sexuality is about universality. Greg McGee says, 'I talk with Tom in colourful scatology describing physical function, as if by reducing it we can understand what drives us.'[39]

Male sexuality in New Zealand might be categorised as an ongoing and intensifying production of sexual sameness and exclusion of sexual difference. The major form of male sexual exclusion in New Zealand, as elsewhere, has been homosexuality. As McNab notes, the socio-economic conditions of early colonial New Zealand meant that people had little time to reflect on or respond to the category 'homosexual'. As a consequence, he argues, 'the emphasis fell on the invisible and the private'.[40] However, the English missionary William Yates's sexuality was the subject of much debate about his sexual relationships with Maori, as was Samuel Butler's long-term relationship with a handsome younger man, Charles Paine Pauli.[41]

Major New Zealand figures such as Frank Sargeson, Charles Brasch and E.H. McCormick, all born in the first decade of the twentieth century, made their mark on the national culture. Growing up during a time of rampant nationalism and through the Great Depression, as Peter Wells states, 'their contribution can be sourced in their own search for personal freedom, arising out of an understanding of the need for social change which would, inter alia, change the conditions under which homosexual men and women lived and suffered'.[42]

Homosexuality was linked with sin and vice from the beginning of colonisation. The early social purity movement was central to the strengthening of the laws against buggery and indecent acts in this country.[43] But buggery, once solely a forbidden act, became transformed over the next fifty years into homosexuality, a category of human perversion, and an abnormal sexual identity. The effect of the proliferation of disparate sexualities meant that there were 'ever more sites where the intensity of pleasures and the persistency of power catch hold',[44] but also that through scientific classification sexual acts between men could be deduced and interpreted, and regulated and cured. By 1949, the discourses of psychiatry had begun to have their impact in New Zealand. The first psychological study of homosexuality in New Zealand reported that six boys who had sexual relationships with older homosexuals became practised liars, were temperamentally unstable, moody, listless and detached, allegedly as a result of their sexual experiences.[45]

Homosexual men suffered intense homophobia, and self-loathing. Bill Logan speaks of his difficulties in coming to terms with his homosexuality: 'I did not want to be gay, I did not want to admit my homosexuality to myself, let alone anyone else .... My homosexuality was there. It wouldn't go away, and I was hating myself for it'.[46] The most shocking New Zealand incident happened in 1964 when five young men were acquitted on charges of manslaughter after going to Hagley Park in Christchurch to look for a homosexual to beat up.

But social change did occur, and in 1985 the Homosexual Law Reform Bill was passed into law, decriminalising sex between men. This change in the law occurred at the intersection of two other momentous events in New Zealand's history: the beginning of the AIDS pandemic, and the 'transformation of the architecture of the state'[47] to a neo-liberal market economy. New modes of sexual governance and conduct came to write themselves on the bodies of gay men. In the New Zealand gay community, bodily pleasure is taking new and different forms, forms regularised by AIDS. The condom, that symbol *par excellence* of regulation of the science of sex, is not only about regulation but about the eroticisation of regulation:

> Like other men of his generation, Gilbert grew up and became sexually active in a world where condoms were associated with erotic pleasure and not sexual health. As he states, 'you used to get all the different varieties of condoms. And they were real play toys you know, all the hot ones that would try to turn you on'. In the last 10 years he had noticed the safer sex and condom messages and used condoms for anal sex with his casual sexual partners.[48]

Homosexual sex, one based around the condom and safe sexual practices in an era of AIDS, prescribes and proscribes, names and categorises sexual acts on a continuum of pleasure and danger. The homosexual body is now normalised and scrutinised.

HEALTH

Modernity is structured on a dependence on life and health. As capitalism requires Brian's productivity and reproductivity, medical and biological sciences take control of his subjectivity and his body. The scientific encroachment of powers on bodies means a growth in classification of disease. The science of life, which Foucault calls bio-power, invests in the body's (re)productive capacity, while anatomo-politics fastens on to the minutiae of the body's functioning, becoming 'embedded in bodies, becoming deeply characteristic, the oddities of sex relied on a technology of health and pathology …'.[49]

While statistical information about men's physical and mental health has generally been readily available in New Zealand, 'men's health' as a sociological construct is a contemporary phenomenon. This conceptualisation has emerged in relation to feminist concerns surrounding 'women's health', and the flourishing writing and interest in masculinities over the past fifteen years. An understanding has evolved from this literature that masculinity is constituted at the intersection of ethnicity, class, sexual preference and physical ability, and that differential access to power is afforded to various masculinities in particular contexts.[50] This theorisation of masculinities as mutable, plural, complex and contradictory is important when thinking about 'men's health' in ways that negate the tendency for sweeping generalisations to mask diversities amongst men.

HIV/AIDS has also incited the formulation of the concept of men's health. Men who have sex with men became the target of health promotion messages encouraging safer sex practices in the mid to late eighties, when it was realised that morbidity rates were escalating amongst this population.[51] In a bid to make these campaigns effective, research was undertaken into sexual behaviour, attitudes towards condoms, and patterns of condom use, in order to determine what put the health of this group 'at risk'.[52] By 1987 public concern about the spread of AIDS into the heterosexual population reached its height, and studies emerged internationally concerning the ways in which the operation of hegemonic masculinities places men at risk for AIDS-related illnesses.[53]

In recent years the media has played a significant role in raising public awareness of specific issues of men's health. A notable example here has been televised coverage of the increasing incidence of prostate and testicular cancer in New Zealand.[54] A documentary screened in 1999 of high-profile television presenter Paul Holmes's battle with this disease brought the daily realities of this cancer into kiwi living-rooms. Similarly, changes to regulations governing the advertisement of prescription drugs on television have made 'Xenical' and 'Viagra' household names. For better or worse, these commercials have made visible the experiences of impotence and clinically diagnosed obesity for men in New Zealand.

Despite the promotion of some aspects of men's health as important within the public arena, it can be argued that the notion of 'taking care of your body' is subordinated amongst other discourses of masculinity and the body. For example, injury within a game of rugby is still commonly constituted as something to endure and 'play through'. This action is constructed as preferable to appearing 'insufficiently masculine' by leaving the field and subsequently letting team-mates down. As Phillips[55] has noted in relation to the All Blacks, the image of the national team has been built on 'pluck and a refusal to admit pain', as epitomised when Norm Hewitt played with a broken arm during the NPC final against Canterbury in 1999.

A MALE HEALTH CRISIS?

A statistic commonly cited in the Western world in relation to the health of men is that their rate of mortality is higher than that of women.[56] For instance, according to latest figures, male mortality continues to exceed female mortality at all ages, with the widest gap in the 15–24 and 25–44 age groups as a consequence of higher male injury (including suicide) at these ages.[57] Prevailing explanations for this phenomenon range from the 'inadequacies' of men's biology to the way in which the operation of masculinity encourages males to engage in behaviours that put their health at greater risk. Typical explanations are:

> Women appear to have greater genetic resistance to infectious diseases, and are also protected by sex hormones from other diseases such as cardiovascular disease. However, this factor is less important than the adverse lifestyle behaviours adopted by males, women's stronger predisposition to seek and continue health care, and the cumulative beneficial effect of extra health care earlier in life for women.[58]

The problem with such explanations of mortality rates is that they lead to an oversimplification of health issues and can potentially feed 'backlash' sentiment about a crisis in men's health.

In fact, in the period since the early 1950s life expectancy for both men and women in New Zealand has increased by 7.00 and 8.12 years respectively: a trend that is expected to continue.[59] There is also evidence to suggest that the gap between women and men's average life expectancy has been narrowing since 1977, due to a decline in male death from heart disease and other causes.[60] While men's life expectancy is not yet quite as long as women's, it is certainly not deteriorating, and its improvement attests to the fact that allegations of a crisis in men's health are unfounded in this respect.

Claims that men experience a health disadvantage in relation to women should also be examined closely. Undoubtedly there are areas of concern for men's health, some of which were identified in a 1996 study undertaken in Auckland and Northland.[61] This report noted that key health issues for men were motor vehicle crashes. This is also supported by national statistics, which indicate that 381 men compared with 156 women died in motor vehicle accidents in 1996.[62]

All of the above issues deserve careful consideration when looking at how gender contributes to such health patterns.[63] A further point is that often studies aimed at uncovering sex differences fail to identify any. For example, women and men were almost equal in the most recent count of mental health admissions in New Zealand.[64] Similarly in Australia, no gender differences were found in health issues as diverse as teenage drug use, age-related prevalence of leg ulcers and glaucoma.[65] What these statistics reveal is the futility of arguments which propose one gender's health is worse than the other: rather, there are areas specific to each which require urgent attention.

Arguments about which gender is more disadvantaged also ignore the diversity which exists within groups of 'men' and 'women'. When this kind of analysis is taken into account, differences between certain clusters of men may be greater than differences between genders. In the 1995/96 policy guidelines for regional health authorities, various groups of men were identified as having particular health and disability needs. These included: men with acute or chronic conditions (including disabilities), men of lower socio-economic status, men whose lifestyle places them at risk, men who have unsafe sex with men, and Maori men and men from Pacific Islands or other ethnic minority groups who correlate with the above categories.[66]

Men who are members of these groups will experience greater risk of various health problems than those who are non-members. This is evidenced in research that indicates Maori male life expectancy at birth was 67.2 years which is eight years less than that for non-Maori males (75.3 years).[67] Similarly, male mortality is also affected by socio-economic status, with a gap of 9.2 years in life expectancy at birth between men living in the least and most deprived regions of New Zealand.[68] What this research tells us is that generalisations about male health disadvantage paint a simplistic view of the differences in health which exist between men, as a result of their ethnicity and social class.

HEALTHY BODIES

The body is often constituted as the primary location of health and its appearance perceived as evidence of healthy behaviour. This has been demonstrated in a study of Scottish men aged between thirty and forty, whose accounts of health were grounded explicitly or implicitly in terms of their own or other's bodies.[69] It is also seen in the images of muscle-rippling men who grace covers of magazines like *Health and Fitness,* offering their bodies as the personification of 'male health'. Good health is equated with the way in which their flesh is a manifestation of strength, power and control – characteristics which are valued within dominant Western conceptions of maleness.

Equating male health with the body might be seen as diverting attention away from other health issues which do not find an easily identifiable physical expression. Certainly the mental health of young men in New Zealand is of serious concern. In 1996, New Zealand had the highest rate of youth suicide amongst OECD countries (Finland, Australia, Canada, USA, Norway, France, Denmark, Sweden, Germany, Japan, UK and Netherlands).[70] Males aged twenty to twenty-four years experienced the highest suicide mortality rate of any age group.[71] Mental health is a less visible issue for men, not only because it is often more difficult to detect as an illness, but because it also implies a vulnerability and 'loss of control' which is damaging to dominant forms of masculinity. Not being able to handle everyday situations or reveal any 'emotional weakness' excludes men from particular contexts. While men's bodies are obviously important, those aspects of their health which have tended to be less visible should not be forgotten.

Despite the centrality of the body to constructions of male health, minimal research has been conducted into men's experience of their bodies in this area or more generally.[72] The research on men's bodies which does exist is concerned with the social discursive constitution of the body. A popular theme here is the examination of the relationship between sport, gender and male bodies and the way in which sporting ideology and discourses of masculinity construct a notion of ideal masculine physicality.[73] Other research describes the ways in which masculinity dictates that males maintain an aloofness towards their bodies, learning to treat them like 'a machine that functions according to its own laws and principles'.[74] Some argue that masculinity operates so as to discourage men from establishing contact with their bodies either by touching or by paying detailed attention to them, so that men do not know their bodies in the way that women are forced to be aware of theirs.[75] This is also the result of unwritten rules that govern the possibilities for men to experience embodiment, such as the 'homosexual connotations' attached to touching or looking at other men. As Phillips has noted in his history of Pakeha masculinity, the rugby field was the only site in which men could physically express their emotions for each other without their actions being construed as 'homosexual'.[76]

These kinds of arguments have given credence to the thesis that 'masculinity is intrinsically damaging' to some men's health and that it is in the interests of men 'to change, abandon or resist aspects of masculinity'.[77] Connell highlights a caveat here, in that, 'It is too easy to produce sweeping statements about the "male role" as a health hazard', statements he says 'which turn out to have more exceptions than applications'.[78] This point refers to that made earlier about the need to acknowledge diversity within masculinities and groups of men, as well as in the health experiences they encounter. What the current literature on men's bodies and health indicates is 'the striking absence of knowledge grounded in the everyday experiences of men themselves'.[79]

THE CONTRIBUTIONS TO THIS BOOK

Bob Connell's keynote speech at the 'Masculinities Conference' forms the first chapter in this book, 'Masculinities and Globalisation', and examines the paradoxical impact of globalisation on masculinity. He argues that in order to understand masculinity on a local level, we must now think in global terms. On one hand, the multiplication of institutions and media mean that masculinities and the power relations inherent in them are constituted in ever more concentrated and standardised forms. On the other, he contends that globalisation and its celebration of difference also allows for new questions to be asked and for the destabilisation of dominant masculine forms.

Unlike Connell's chapter, which focuses on the global, that by Park *et al.* examines the local specificities of Samoan masculinity. 'A Late Twentieth-Century Auckland Perspective on Samoan Masculinities' examines the relation of sex/gender and kinship to masculinity and to Samoan men's roles and responsibilities in reproduction, contrasting older and younger men. Using a model developed earlier by anthropologist Bradd Shore, the authors found that generational change occurred between older and younger men. Young men had increasingly flexible gender performances. They carried out 'feminine' domestic chores that older men did not, and sexual fidelity was more important to them than to their older counterparts. However, the key role of economic provider was strongly emphasised by both groups.

Throughout this introduction, we have referred to the importance of rugby in defining New Zealand manhood. Richard Pringle examines his childhood experiences of rugby and masculinity in his chapter, 'Living the Contradictions: a Foucauldian examination of my youth rugby experiences'. He contends that dominating discourses of masculinity associated with rugby shaped his subjectivity in complex ways. The pain and violence that Pringle experienced on the rugby field made him question the place of rugby in his life.

While Pringle examines what might be the hegemonic constitution of masculinity through rugby, Terry O'Neill's chapter 'Managing the Margins: gay-disabled masculinity' discusses the problem of being a gay and disabled man in New Zealand. For O'Neill, the conjunction of homosexuality and disability brings a sense of difference. He says, 'gay-disabled [masculinity is an] … ambiguous sensibility and discursive articulation of the ways in which non-hegemonic males are understood by themselves and others to be maintained in relation to power'.

Clive Aspin's chapter, 'I didn't have to go to finishing school to learn how to be gay: Maori gay men's understanding of cultural and sexual identity', draws on historical sources to contextualise his discussion. He argues that current Maori masculinities are informed by both traditional Maori and colonial forms. Gay Maori men 'draw considerable strength and inspiration from the knowledge that the word *takatapui* existed within pre-European society'. Nowadays, *takatapui* have to come to terms with their own multiple identities (as both gay and Maori) and with the claims made by each.

Masculinity can be a very fluid concept, as Heather Worth discusses in her chapter, 'Tits is Just an Accessory: South Auckland queens and masculinity'. She argues that Maori and Pacific queens think of themselves in ways which are inimical to a Western view that we must be one sex or the other, or that we must choose a stable gender. For these queens, gender and sexual identity involve both masculinity and femininity.

Annie Potts' chapter, 'The Man with Two Brains: the discursive construction of the unreasonable penis-self', unpacks the ways in which kiwi men and women discuss the penis in terms of spatial tropes: 'the relationship between the man and his penis is complex: while the man's body may be envisaged as external to his self, the penis stands apart form the man. Often this leads to a battle of wills – when the penis has a "mind" of its own'. Consequently, Potts argues, men dissociate their penis from themselves during sex and thus absolve themselves from any sexual responsibility.

In contrast, Louisa Allen's chapter, 'As far as sex goes I don't really think about my body: young men's corporeal experiences of (hetero)sexual pleasure', examines both young men's sexual disembodiment, and also the intense care and surveillance of their bodies. For the men in her study, the 'feelings of dissatisfaction with bodies, revealed a negative relationship distorted by dominant perceptions of masculine bodily perfection'. Allen found that being in an emotional relationship allowed these young men to experience a bodily sensuality beyond the limits of hegemonic sexuality.

The models and practices of masculinity affect the way young New Zealand men think about their health. In 'Young Pakeha Men's Conceptions of Health and Illness', Anthony O'Connor argues that demonstrating control over one's body means that one can ignore signs of ill-health and not go to the doctor. There is much to discourage men from taking care of their health: 'there is a negotiation required to strike a balance between health status, masculinity and the social setting which on many occasions position masculinity and health care in conflict'.

In the final chapter, 'Abducted by Aliens: heterosexual men and sexual health', Stephen McKernon discusses the experiences of heterosexual men of a sexual health service and the challenge sexual health poses to masculinity. The sexuality of heterosexual men has been silenced in sexual health programmes and policies. McKernon's research suggests that kiwi heterosexual men feel sex is stigmatised to the degree that they have incomplete knowledge and as adults need information and advice on sexual health matters.

one

Masculinities and Globalisation

R.W. CONNELL

The current wave of research and debate on masculinity stems from the impact of the women's liberation movement on men; but it has taken time for this impact to produce a new intellectual agenda. Most discussions of men's gender in the 1970s and early 1980s centred on an established concept: the 'male sex role', and an established problem: how men and boys were 'socialised' into this role. There was not much new empirical research. What there was tended to use the more abstracted methods of social psychology (e.g. paper-and-pencil masculinity/femininity scales) to measure generalised attitudes and expectations in ill-defined populations. The largest body of empirical research was the continuing stream of quantitative studies of sex differences – which continued to be disappointingly slight.[1]

The concept of a unitary male 'sex role', however, came under increasing criticism for its multiple oversimplifications and its incapacity to handle issues about power.[2] New conceptual frameworks were proposed, which linked feminist work on institutionalised patriarchy, gay theoretical work on homophobia, and psychoanalytic ideas about the person.[3] Increasing attention was given to certain studies which located issues about masculinity in a fully described local context, whether a British printing shop[4] or a Papuan mountain community.[5] By the late 1980s a genre of empirical research based on these ideas was developing, most clearly in sociology but also in anthropology, history, organisation studies and cultural studies. This has borne fruit in the 1990s in what is now widely recognised as a new generation of social research on masculinity and men in gender relations.[6]

Though the recent research has been diverse in subject-matter and social location, its characteristic focus is the construction of masculinity in a particular milieu or moment – a clergyman's family,[7] a professional sports career,[8] a small group of gay men,[9] a bodybuilding gym,[10] a group of colonial schools,[11] an urban police force,[12] drinking groups in bars,[13] a corporate office on the verge of a decision.[14] Accordingly we might think of this as the 'ethnographic moment' in masculinity research, in which the specific and the local is in focus.

(This is not to deny that this work *deploys* broader structural concepts, but simply to note the characteristic focus of the empirical work and its analysis).

The ethnographic moment brought a much-needed gust of realism to debates on men and masculinity, a corrective to the simplifications of role theory. It also provided a corrective to the trend in popular culture where vague discussions of men's sex roles were giving way to the mystical generalities of the 'mythopoetic' movement and the extreme simplifications of religious revivalism. Though the rich detail of the historical and field studies defies easy summary, certain conclusions emerge from this body of research as a whole. These are summarised under the following subheadings:

Plural masculinities

A theme of theoretical work in the 1980s, the multiplicity of masculinities, has now been very fully documented by descriptive research. Different cultures, and different periods of history, construct gender differently. Striking differences exist, for instance, in the relationship of homosexual practice to dominant forms of masculinity.[15] In multicultural societies there are varying definitions and enactments of masculinity, for instance between Anglo and Latin communities in the United States.[16] Equally important, more than one kind of masculinity can be found within a given cultural setting or institution. This is particularly well documented in school studies[17] but can also be observed in workplaces[18] and the military.[19]

Hierarchy and hegemony

Plural masculinities exist in definite social relations, often relations of hierarchy and exclusion. This was recognised early, in gay theorists' discussions of homophobia; it has become clear that the implications are far-reaching. There is generally a 'hegemonic' form of masculinity: the most honoured or desired in a particular context. For Western popular culture, this is extensively documented in research on media representations of masculinity.[20] The hegemonic form, however, is not necessarily the most common form of masculinity. Many men live in a state of some tension with, or distance from, hegemonic masculinity; others (such as sporting heroes) are taken as exemplars of hegemonic masculinity and are fully expected to live up to it.[21] The dominance of hegemonic masculinity over other forms may be quiet and implicit, but may also be vehement and brutal, as in homophobic violence.

Collective masculinities

Masculinities, as patterns of gender practice, are sustained and enacted not only by individuals, but also by groups and institutions. This fact was visible in Cockburn's pioneering research on informal workplace culture,[22] and has been confirmed over and over: in workplaces,[23] in organised sport,[24] in schools[25] and elsewhere. This conclusion must be taken with the previous two: institutions may construct multiple masculinities and define relationships between them. Barrett's illuminating study of hegemonic masculinity in the US Navy shows how this takes different forms in the different sub-branches of the one military organisation.[26]

Bodies as arenas

Men's bodies do not determine the patterns of masculinity, but they are still of great importance in masculinity. Men's bodies are addressed, defined and disciplined (as in sport),[27] and given outlets and pleasures by the gender order of society. But men's bodies are not blank slates. The enactment of masculinity reaches certain limits, for instance in the destruction of the industrial worker's body.[28] Masculine conduct with a female body is felt to be anomalous or transgressive, like feminine conduct with a male body; research on gender crossing shows the work that must be done to sustain an anomalous gender.[29]

Active construction

Masculinities do not exist prior to social interaction, but come into existence as people act. They are actively produced, using the resources and strategies available in a given milieu. Thus the exemplary masculinities of sports professionals are not a product of passive disciplining, but as Messner shows, result from a sustained, active engagement with the demands of the institutional setting, even to the point of serious bodily damage from 'playing hurt' and accumulated stress.[30] With boys learning masculinities, much of what was previously taken as 'socialisation' appears, in close-focus studies of schools,[31] as the outcome of intricate and intense manoeuvring in peer groups, classes and adult-child relationships.

Contradiction

Masculinities are not homogeneous, simple states of being. Close-focus research on masculinities commonly identifies contradictory desires and conduct; for instance, in Klein's study of bodybuilders, between the heterosexual definition of hegemonic masculinity and the homosexual practice through which some of the group he studied financed the making of an exemplary body.[32] Psychoanalysis provides the classic evidence of conflicts within personality, and recent psychoanalytic writing has laid some emphasis on the conflicts and emotional compromises within both hegemonic and subordinated forms of masculinity.[33] Life-history research influenced by existential psychoanalysis has similarly traced contradictory projects and commitments within particular forms of masculinity.[34]

Dynamics

Masculinities created in specific historical circumstances are liable to reconstruction, and any pattern of hegemony is subject to contestation in which a dominant masculinity may be displaced. Heward shows the changing gender regime of a boys' school responding to the changed strategies of the families in its clientele.[35] Roper shows the displacement of a production-oriented masculinity among engineering managers by new financially oriented generic managers.[36] Since the 1970s the reconstruction of masculinities has been pursued as a conscious politics. Schwalbe's close examination of one mythopoetic group shows the complexity of the practice and the limits of the reconstruction.[37]

If we compare this picture of masculinity with earlier understandings of the 'male sex role', it is clear that the ethnographic moment in research has already had important intellectual fruits. Nevertheless, it has always been recognised that some issues go beyond the local. For instance, the mythopoetic movement, like the highly visible Promise Keepers, are part of a spectrum of masculinity politics; Messner shows for the United States that this spectrum involves at least eight conflicting agendas for the remaking of masculinity.[38] Historical studies such as Phillips[39] on New Zealand and Kimmel[40] on the United States have traced the changing public constructions of masculinity for whole countries over long periods; ultimately, such historical reconstructions are essential for understanding the meaning of ethnographic details.

I consider that this logic must now be taken a step further; and in taking this step, we will move towards a new agenda for the whole field. What happens in localities is affected by the history of whole countries, but what happens in countries is affected by the history of the world. Locally situated lives are now (indeed, have long been) powerfully influenced by geopolitical struggles, global markets, multinational corporations, labour migration, transnational media. It is time for this fundamental fact to be built into our analysis of men and masculinities.

To understand local masculinities, we must think in global terms. But how? That is the problem pursued in this essay. I will offer a framework for thinking about masculinities as a feature of world society, and for thinking about men's gender practices in terms of the global structure and dynamics of gender. This is by no means to reject the 'ethnographic moment' in masculinity research. It is, rather, to think about how we can use its findings more adequately.

The world gender order

Masculinities do not first exist, and then come into contact with femininities; they are produced together, in the process that constitutes a gender order. Accordingly, to understand the masculinities on a world scale we must first have a concept of the globalisation of gender. This is one of the most difficult points in current gender analysis because the very conception is counter-intuitive. We are so accustomed to thinking of gender as the attribute of an individual – even as an unusually intimate attribute – that it requires a considerable wrench to think of gender on the vast scale of global society. Most relevant discussions, such as the literature on 'women and development', fudge the issue. They treat the entities that extend internationally (markets, corporations, intergovernmental programmes) as ungendered in principle – but impacting unequally on gendered recipients of aid in practice, because of bad policies. Such conceptions reproduce the familiar liberal-feminist view of the state as in principle gender-neutral, though empirically dominated by men.

But if we recognise that very large-scale institutions, such as the state, are themselves gendered in quite precise and specifiable ways,[41] and if we recognise that international relations, international trade and global markets are inherently an arena of gender formation and gender politics,[42] then we can recognise the existence of a world gender order. The term can be defined as the structure of relationships that interconnect the gender regimes of institutions, and the gender orders of local society, on a world scale. That is, however, only a definition. The substantive questions remain: what is the shape of that structure, how tightly are its elements linked, how has it arisen historically, and what is its trajectory into the future.

Current business and media talk about 'globalisation' pictures a homogenising process sweeping across the world, driven by new technologies, producing vast, unfettered global markets in which all participate on equal terms. This is a misleading image. As Hirst and Thompson show, the global economy is highly unequal and the current degree of homogenisation is often overestimated.[43] Multinational corporations based in the three major economic powers (the United States, European Union, and Japan) are the major economic actors worldwide.

The structure bears the marks of its history. Modern global society was historically produced, as Wallerstein argued, by the economic and political expansion of European states from the fifteenth century on, and by the creation of colonial empires.[44] It is in this process that we find the roots of the modern world gender order. Imperialism was, from the start, a gendered process. Its first phase, colonial conquest and settlement, was carried out by gender-segregated forces, and resulted in massive disruption of indigenous gender orders. In its second phase, the stabilisation of colonial societies, new gender divisions of labour were produced in plantation economies and colonial cities, while gender ideologies were linked with racial hierarchies and the cultural defence of empire. The third phase, marked by political decolonisation, economic neocolonialism, and the current growth of world markets and structures of financial control, has seen gender divisions of labour remade on a massive scale in the 'global factory',[45] as well as the spread of gendered violence alongside Western military technology. The result of this history is a partially integrated, highly unequal and turbulent world society, in which gender relations are partly but unevenly linked on a global scale. The unevenness becomes clear when different substructures of gender, identified by the subheadings below, are examined separately.[46]

The division of labour

A characteristic feature of colonial and neocolonial economies was the restructuring of local production systems to produce a couple consisting of a male wage-worker and a female domestic-worker.[47] This need not produce a 'housewife' in the Western suburban sense, for instance where the waged work involved migration to plantations or mines.[48] But it has generally produced the identification of masculinity with the public realm and the money economy, and of femininity with domesticity, that is a core feature of the modern European gender system.[49]

Power relations

The colonial and postcolonial world has tended to break down purdah systems of patriarchy in the name of modernisation, if not of women's emancipation.[50] At the same time, the creation of a westernised public realm has seen the growth of large-scale organisations in the form of the state and corporations, which are almost always culturally masculinised, and controlled by men. In 'comprador' capitalism, however, the power of local élites depends on their relations with the metropolitan powers, so the hegemonic masculinities of neocolonial societies are uneasily poised between local and global cultures.

Emotional relations

Both religious and cultural 'missionary' activity has corroded indigenous homosexual and cross-gender practice, such as the native American 'berdache' and the Chinese 'passion of the cut sleeve'.[51] Recently developed Western models of romantic heterosexual love leading to marriage, and of gay identity as the main alternative, have now circulated globally – though as Altman observes, they do not simply displace indigenous models, but interact with them in extremely complex ways.[52]

Symbolisation

Mass media, especially electronic media, in most parts of the world follow North American and European models and relay a great deal of metropolitan content; gender imagery is an important part of what is circulated. A striking example is the reproduction of a North American image of femininity by Xuxa, the blonde television superstar in Brazil.[53] In counterpoint, 'exotic' gender imagery has been used in the marketing strategies of newly industrialising countries (e.g. airline advertising from South-East Asia) – a tactic based on knowledge of the longstanding combination of the exotic and the erotic that appeals to the colonial imagination.[54]

Clearly, the world gender order is not simply an extension of a traditional European-American gender order. That gender order was changed by colonialism, and elements from other cultures now circulate globally. Yet in no sense do they mix on equal terms, to produce a United Colours of Benetton gender order. The culture and institutions of the North Atlantic countries are hegemonic within the emergent world system. Awareness of this is crucial for understanding the kinds of masculinities produced within it.

The repositioning of men and the reconstitution of masculinities

The positioning of men and the constitution of masculinities may be analysed at any of the levels at which gender practice is configured: in relation to the body, in personal life and in collective social practice. At each level we need to consider how the processes of globalisation influence configurations of gender.

Men's bodies are positioned in the gender order, and enter the gender process, through body-reflexive practices in which bodies are both objects and agents[55] – including sexuality, violence and labour. The conditions of such practices include where one is, and who is available for interaction. So it is a fact of considerable importance for gender relations that the global social order distributes and redistributes bodies – through migration, and through political controls over movement and interaction.

The creation of empire was the original 'élite migration', though in certain instances mass migration followed. Through settler colonialism, something close to the gender order of Western Europe was reassembled in North America and in Australasia. Labour migration within the colonial systems was a means by which gender practices were spread, but also a means by which they were reconstructed, since labour migration was itself a gendered process – as we have seen in relation to the gender division of labour. Migration from the colonised world to the metropole became (except for Japan) a mass process in the decades after the Second World War. There is also migration within the periphery, such as the creation of a very large immigrant labour force, mostly from other Muslim countries, into the oil-producing Gulf states.

These relocations of bodies create the possibility of hybridisation in gender imagery and sexuality, and in other forms of practice. The movement is not always towards synthesis, however, as the racial and ethnic hierarchies of colonialism have been recreated in new contexts, including the politics of the metropole. Ethnic and racial conflict has been growing in importance in recent years, and as Klein and Tillner argue, this context is likely to produce masculinities oriented towards domination and violence.[56] Even without the context of violence, there can be an intimate interweaving of the formation of masculinity with the formation of ethnic identity, as seen in the study by Poynting *et al.* of Lebanese youth in the Anglo-dominant culture of Australia.[57]

At the level of personal life as well as in relation to bodies, the making of masculinities is shaped by global forces. Sometimes the link is indirect, as is seen in the example of working-class Australian men caught in a situation of structural unemployment which arises from Australia's changing position in the global economy.[58] At other times the link is obvious, such as that between the executives of multinational corporations and the financial sector servicing international trade. The requirements of a career in international business set up strong pressures on domestic life: almost all multinational executives are men, and the assumption in business magazines and advertising directed towards them is that they will have a dependent wife running their home and bringing up their children.

At the level of collective practice, masculinities are reconstituted by the remaking of gender meanings, and the reshaping of the institutional contexts of practice. Let us consider each in turn.

The growth of global mass media, especially electronic media, is an obvious 'vector' for the globalisation of gender. Popular entertainment circulates stereotyped gender images, deliberately made attractive for marketing purposes. The example of Xuxa in Brazil has already been mentioned. International news media are also controlled or strongly influenced from the metropole, and circulate Western definitions of authoritative masculinity, criminality, desirable femininity and other cultural stereotypes. But there are limits to the power of global mass communications. Some local centres of mass entertainment differ from the Hollywood model, such as the Indian popular film industry centred in Bombay. Further, media research emphasises that audiences are highly selective in their reception of media messages, and we must allow for popular recognition of the fantasy in mass entertainment. Just as economic globalisation can be exaggerated, the creation of a 'global culture' is a more turbulent and uneven process than is often assumed.[59]

More important, I would argue, is a process that began long before electronic media existed in the export of institutions. Gendered institutions not only circulate definitions of masculinity (and femininity), as sex-role theory notes. The functioning of gendered institutions, creating specific conditions for social practice, calls into existence specific patterns of practice. Thus, certain patterns of collective violence are embedded in the organisation and culture of a Western-style army, which are different from the patterns of violence in pre-colonial societies. Certain patterns of calculative egocentrism are embedded in the working of a stock market; certain patterns of rule-following and domination are embedded in a bureaucracy.

The colonial and postcolonial world has seen the installation in the periphery, on a very large scale, of a range of institutions on the North Atlantic model: armies, states, bureaucracies, corporations, capital markets, labour markets, schools, law courts, transport systems. These are gendered institutions, and their functioning has directly reconstituted masculinities in the periphery. This has not necessarily meant Xerox copies of European masculinities. Rather, pressures for change, inherent in the institutional form, are set up.

To the extent particular institutions become dominant in world society, the patterns of masculinity embedded in them may become global standards. Masculine dress is an interesting indicator: almost every political leader in the world now wears the uniform of the Western business executive. The more common pattern, however, is not the complete displacement of local patterns but the articulation of the local gender order with the gender regime of global-model institutions. Case studies such as Hollway's account of bureaucracy in Tanzania illustrate the point: there, domestic patriarchy articulated with masculine authority in the state, in ways that subverted the government's formal commitment to equal opportunity for women.[60]

We should not expect the overall structure of gender relations on a world scale simply to mirror patterns known on the smaller scale. In the most vital of respects there is continuity. The world gender order is unquestionably patriarchal, in the sense that it privileges men over women. There is a 'patriarchal dividend' for men arising from unequal wages, unequal labour force participation, and a highly unequal structure of ownership, as well as cultural and sexual privileging. This has been extensively documented by feminist work, done mainly in the 1980s, on women's situation globally,[61] though its implications for masculinity have mostly been ignored. The conditions thus exist for the production of a hegemonic masculinity on a world scale: that is to say, a dominant form of masculinity which embodies, organises and legitimates men's domination in the gender order as a whole.

The conditions of globalisation, which involve the interaction of many local gender orders, certainly multiply the forms of masculinity in the global gender order. At the same time, the specific shape of globalisation, concentrating economic and cultural power on an unprecedented scale, provide new resources for dominance by particular groups of men. This dominance may become institutionalised in a pattern of masculinity which becomes, to some degree, standardised across localities. I will call such patterns 'globalising masculinities', and it is among them, rather than narrowly within the metropole, that we are likely to find candidates for hegemony in the world gender order.

Globalising masculinities

In this section I will offer a sketch of major forms of globalising masculinity, in the three historical phases identified above in the discussion of globalisation.

Masculinities of conquest and settlement

The creation of the imperial social order involved peculiar conditions for the gender practices of men. Colonial conquest itself was mainly carried out by segregated groups of men – soldiers, sailors, traders, administrators, and a good many who were all these by turn (such as the 'Rum Corps' in early New South Wales). They came from the more segregated occupations and milieux in the metropole, and it is likely that the men drawn into colonisation tended to be the more rootless of them. Certainly the process of conquest could produce frontier masculinities which combined the occupational culture of these groups with an unusual level of violence and egocentric individualism. The vehement contemporary debate about the genocidal violence of the Spanish conquistadors – who in fifty years completely exterminated the population of Hispaniola – points to this pattern.[62]

The political history of empire is full of evidence of the tenuous control over the frontier exercised by the state – the Spanish monarchs unable to rein in the conquistadors, the governors in Sydney unable to hold back the squatters and in Capetown unable to hold back the Boers, gold rushes breaking boundaries everywhere, even an independent republic set up by escaped slaves in Brazil. The point probably applies to other forms of social control too, such as customary controls on men's sexuality. Extensive sexual exploitation of indigenous women was a common feature of conquest. In certain circumstances frontier masculinities might be reproduced as a local cultural tradition long after the frontier had passed, such as the gauchos of southern South America, the cowboys of the western USA.

In other circumstances, however, the frontier of conquest and exploitation was replaced by a frontier of settlement. Sex ratios in the colonising population changed, as women arrived and locally born generations succeeded. A shift back towards the family patterns of the metropole was likely. As Cain and Hopkins have shown for the British empire, the ruling group in the colonial world as a whole was an extension of the dominant class in the metropole – the landed gentry – and tended to reproduce its social customs and ideology.[63] The creation of a settler masculinity might be the goal of state policy, as it seems to have been in late nineteenth-century New Zealand, as part of a general process of pacification and the creation of an agricultural social order.[64] Or it might be undertaken through institutions created by settler groups, such as the élite schools in Natal studied by Morrell.[65]

The impact of colonialism on the construction of masculinity among the colonised is much less documented, but there is every reason to think it was severe. Conquest and settlement disrupted all the structures of indigenous society, whether or not this was intended by the colonising powers.[66] Indigenous gender orders were no exception. Their disruption could result from the pulverisation of indigenous communities (as in the seizure of land in eastern North America and southeastern Australia), through gendered labour migration (as in goldmining with black labour in South Africa),[67] to ideological attacks on local gender arrangements (as in the missionary assault on the 'berdache' tradition in North America).[68] The varied course of resistance to colonisation is also likely to have affected the making of masculinities. This is clear in the region of Natal in South Africa, where sustained resistance to colonisation by the Zulu kingdom was a key to the mobilisation of ethnic-national masculine identities in the twentieth century.[69]

Masculinities of empire

The imperial social order created a hierarchy of masculinities, as it created a hierarchy of communities and races. The colonisers distinguished 'more manly' from 'less manly' groups among their subjects. In British India, for instance, Bengali men were supposed effeminate while Pathans and Sikhs were regarded as strong and warlike. Similar distinctions were made in South Africa between 'Hottentots' and Zulus, in North America between Iroquois, Sioux and Cheyenne on one side and southern and southwestern tribes on the other.

At the same time, the emerging imagery of gender difference in European culture provided general symbols of superiority and inferiority. Within the imperial 'poetics of war', the conqueror was virile, while the colonised were dirty, sexualised, and effeminate or childlike.[70] In many colonial situations indigenous men were called 'boys' by the colonisers (e.g. in Zimbabwe).[71] Sinha's interesting study of the language of political controversy in India in the 1880s and 1890s shows how the images of 'manly Englishman' and 'effeminate Bengali' were deployed to uphold colonial privilege and contain movements for change.[72] In the late nineteenth century, racial barriers in colonial societies were hardening rather than weakening, and gender ideology tended to fuse with racism in forms that the twentieth century never untangled.

The power relations of empire meant that indigenous gender orders were generally under pressure from the colonisers, rather than the other way around. But the colonisers too might change. The barriers of late colonial racism were not only to prevent pollution from below, but also to forestall 'going native', a well-recognised possibility – the starting-point, for instance, of Kipling's famous novel *Kim*.[73] In addition, the pressures, opportunities and profits of empire might work changes in gender arrangements among the colonisers, for instance the division of labour in households with a large supply of indigenous workers as domestic servants.[74] Furthermore, empire might affect the gender order of the metropole itself: through changing gender ideologies, divisions of labour, and the nature of the metropolitan state. For instance, empire figured prominently as a source of masculine imagery in Britain, in the Boy Scouts and in the cult of Lawrence of Arabia.[75] Here we see examples of an important principle: the *interplay* of gender dynamics between different parts of the world order.

The world of empire created two very different settings for the modernisation of masculinities. In the periphery, the forcible restructuring of economies and work forces tended to individualise, on the one hand, and rationalise on the other. A widespread result was masculinities in which the rational calculation of self-interest was the key to action, emphasising the European gender contrast of rational man/irrational woman. The specific form might be local – for instance the Japanese 'salaryman', a type first recognised in the 1910s, was specific to the Japanese context of large, stable industrial conglomerates.[76] But the result generally was masculinities defined around economic action, with both workers and entrepreneurs increasingly adapting to emerging market economies.

In the metropole, the accumulation of wealth made possible a specialisation of leadership in the dominant classes, and struggles for hegemony in which masculinities organised around domination or violence were split from masculinities organised around expertise. The class compromises that allowed the development of the welfare state in Europe and North America were paralleled by gender compromises – gender reform movements (most notably the women's suffrage movement) contesting the legal privileges of men and forcing concessions from the state. In this context, agendas of reform in masculinity emerged: the temperance movement, companionate marriage, homosexual rights movements, leading eventually to the pursuit of 'androgyny' in 'men's liberation' in the 1970s.[77] Not all reconstructions of masculinity, however, emphasised tolerance or moved towards androgyny. The vehement masculinity politics of fascism, for instance, emphasised dominance and difference, and glorified violence, a pattern still found in contemporary racist movements.[78]

Masculinities of postcolonialism and neoliberalism

The process of decolonisation disrupted the gender hierarchies of the colonial order, and where armed struggle was involved, at times involved a deliberate cultivation of masculine hardness and violence (as in South Africa).[79] Some activists and theorists of liberation struggles celebrated this, as a necessary response to colonial violence and emasculation; women in liberation struggles were perhaps less impressed. However one evaluates the process, one of the consequences of decolonisation was another round of disruptions of community-based gender orders, and another step in the reorientation of masculinities towards national and international contexts.

Nearly half a century after the main wave of decolonisation, the old hierarchies persist in new shapes. With the collapse of Soviet communism, the decline of postcolonial socialism, and the ascendancy of the new right in Europe and North America, world politics is more and more organised around the needs of transnational capital and the creation of global markets.

The neoliberal agenda has little to say, explicitly, about gender: it speaks a gender-neutral language of 'markets', 'individuals', and 'choice'. But the world in which neoliberalism is ascendant is still a gendered world, and neoliberalism has an implicit gender politics. The 'individual' of neoliberal theory has in general the attributes and interests of a male entrepreneur, the attack on the welfare state generally weakens the position of women, while the increasingly unregulated power of transnational corporations places strategic power in the hands of particular groups of men. It is not surprising, then, that the installation of capitalism in Eastern Europe and the former Soviet Union has been accompanied by a reassertion of dominating masculinities and, in some situations, a sharp worsening in the social position of women.

We might propose, then, that the hegemonic form of masculinity in the current world gender order is the masculinity associated with those who control its dominant institutions: the business executives who operate in global markets, and the political executives who interact (and in many contexts merge) with them. I will call this 'transnational business masculinity'. This is not readily available for ethnographic study, but we can get some clues to its character from its reflections in management literature, business journalism, corporate self-promotion, and from studies of local business élites.[80]

As a first approximation I would suggest this is a masculinity marked by increasing egocentrism, very conditional loyalties (even to the corporation), and a declining sense of responsibility for others (except for purposes of image-making). Gee *et al.*, studying recent management textbooks, note the peculiar construction of the executive in 'fast capitalism' as a person with no permanent commitments, except (in effect) to the idea of accumulation itself.[81] Transnational business masculinity is characterised by a limited technical rationality ('management theory') which is increasingly separate from science.

Transnational business masculinity differs from traditional bourgeois masculinity by its increasingly libertarian sexuality, with a growing tendency to commodify relations with women. Hotels catering for businessmen in most parts of the world now routinely offer pornographic videos, and in some parts of the world there is a well-developed prostitution industry catering for international businessmen. Transnational business masculinity does not require a powerful physique, since the patriarchal dividend on which it rests is accumulated by impersonal, institutional means. But corporations increasingly use images of the exemplary bodies of élite sportsmen as a marketing tool (as seen in the exceptional growth of corporate 'sponsorship' of sport in the last generation), and indirectly as a means of legitimation for the whole global gender order.

Masculinity politics on a world scale

Recognising global society as an arena of masculinity formation allows us to pose new questions about masculinity politics. What social dynamics in the global arena give rise to masculinity politics, and what shape does global masculinity politics take?

The gradual creation of a world gender order has meant many local instabilities of gender. Gender instability is a familiar theme of poststructuralist theory, but this school of thought takes as a universal condition a situation that is historically specific. Instabilities range, for example, from the disruption of men's local cultural dominance as women move into the public realm and higher education, through the disruption of sexual identities that produced 'queer' politics in the metropole, to the shifts in the urban intelligentsia that produced 'the new-age sensitive guy' and other images of gender change.

One response to such instabilities, on the part of groups whose power is challenged but still dominant, is to reaffirm *local* gender orthodoxies and hierarchies. A masculine fundamentalism is, accordingly, a common response in gender politics at present. A soft version, searching for an essential masculinity among myths and symbols, is offered by the 'mythopoetic' men's movement in the United States, and by the religious revivalists of the Promise Keepers.[82] A much harder version is found, in that country, in the right-wing militia movement brought to world attention by the Oklahoma City bombing;[83] and in contemporary Afghanistan, if we can trust Western media reports, in the militant misogyny of the Talibaan. It is no coincidence that in the two latter cases, hardline masculine fundamentalism goes together with a marked anti-internationalism. The world system – rightly enough – is seen as the source of pollution and disruption.

Not that the emerging global order is a hotbed of gender progressivism. Indeed, the neoliberal agenda for the reform of national and international economies involves closing down historic possibilities for gender reform. I have noted how it subverts the gender compromise represented by the metropolitan welfare state. It has also undermined the progressive-liberal agendas of sex-role reform represented by affirmative action programmes, anti-discrimination provisions, childcare services, and the like. Right-wing parties and governments have been persistently cutting such programmes, in the name either of individual liberties or global competitiveness. Through these means the patriarchal dividend to men is defended or restored, without an *explicit* masculinity politics in the form of a mobilisation of men.

Within the arenas of international relations, the international state, multinational corporations and global markets, there is nevertheless a deployment of masculinities and a reasonably clear hegemony. The transnational business masculinity described above has had only one major competitor for hegemony in recent decades: the rigid, control-oriented masculinity of the military, and the military-style bureaucratic dictatorships of Stalinism. With the collapse of Stalinism and the end of the cold war, Big Brother (Orwell's famous parody of this form of masculinity) is a fading threat, and the more flexible, calculative, egocentric masculinity of the 'fast capitalist' entrepreneur holds the world stage.

We must, however, recall two important conclusions of the ethnographic moment in masculinity research: that different forms of masculinity exist together, and that hegemony is constantly subject to challenge. These are possibilities in the global arena too. Transnational business masculinity is not completely homogeneous; variations of it are embedded in different parts of the world-system, which may not be completely compatible. We may distinguish a Confucian variant, based in East Asia, with a stronger commitment to hierarchy and social consensus, from a secularised-Christian variant, based in North America, with more hedonism and individualism, and greater tolerance for social conflict. In certain arenas there is already conflict between the business and political leaderships embodying these forms of masculinity: initially over 'human rights' versus 'Asian values', and more recently over the extent of trade and investment liberalisation.

If these are contenders for hegemony, there is also the possibility of opposition to hegemony. The global circulation of 'gay' identity is an important indication that non-hegemonic masculinities may operate in global arenas,[84] and may even find a certain political articulation, in this case around human rights and AIDS prevention.

Critiques of dominant forms of masculinity have been circulating for some time among heterosexual men, or among groups which are predominantly heterosexual. English-language readers will be most familiar with three Anglophone examples: the 'anti-sexist' or 'pro-feminist' men's groups in the United States, with their umbrella group NOMAS (National Organization of Men Against Sexism) which has been running since the early 1980s;[85] the British new left men's groups, which produced the remarkable magazine *Achilles Heel*;[86] and the Canadian 'White Ribbon' campaign, the most successful mass mobilisation of men opposing men's violence against women.[87]

There are parallel developments in other language communities. In Germany, for instance, feminists launched a discussion of the gender of men in the 1980s,[88] which has been followed by an educational,[89] a popular-psychology[90] and a critical[91] debate about masculinities and how to change them. In Scandinavia, gender reform has led to the 'father's quota' of parental leave in Norway[92] and to a particularly active network of masculinity researchers. In Japan, a media debate about 'men's liberation', and some pioneering books about changing masculinities,[93] have been followed by the foundation of a men's centre and diversifying debates on change.

These developments at national or regional level have, very recently, begun to link internationally. An International Association for Studies of Men has begun to link men involved in critical studies of masculinity. Certain international agencies, including UNESCO,[94] have sponsored conferences to discuss the policy implications of new perspectives on masculinity.

Compared with the concentration of institutional power in multinational businesses, these initiatives remain small-scale and dispersed. They are, nevertheless, important in potential. I have argued that the global gender order contains, necessarily, greater plurality of gender forms than any local gender order. This must reinforce the consciousness that masculinity is not one fixed form. The plurality of masculinities, at least symbolically, prefigures the unconstrained creativity of a democratic gender order.

Concluding note

If the perspective set out in this chapter holds good, it suggests a significant refocusing of the research agenda on masculinities. There is already a move beyond strictly local studies in the direction of comparative studies from different parts of the world.[95] My argument suggests moving beyond this again, to study of the global arena itself, both as a venue for the social construction of masculinities, and as a powerful force in local gender dynamics. Such a move will require a reconsideration of research methods, since the life-history and ethnographic methods that have been central to recent work on masculinities give limited grasp on the very large-scale institutions, markets, and mass communications that are in play on the world stage. Finally, the typical researcher of recent years – the individual scholar with a personal research project – will need to be supplemented by international teams, able to work together for significant periods, to investigate issues of the scale and complexity we must now address.

two

Late Twentieth-Century Auckland Perspective on Samoan Masculinities

Julie Park, Tamasailau Suaalii-Sauni, Melani Anae, Ieti Lima, Nite Fuamatu and Kirk Mariner

Nearly twenty years ago an anthropologist of island Samoa, Bradd Shore, summed up his own and other scholars' perceptions of the Samoan sex/gender matrix by contrasting the relative lack of social attention to male sexuality compared with great attention to female sexuality, and the relative focus of attention on male gender behaviour compared with the lack of attention to female gender behaviour.[1] His formulation coincides with that of other contemporary scholars.[2] Our purpose is to use this model, derived in island Samoa more than twenty years ago, to examine Samoan men's roles and responsibilities in reproduction in Auckland, at the end of the twentieth century.

Sex and gender in the Samoa context

Shore distinguishes reproductive sexuality from, on the one hand, psychological sexuality, and, on the other, gender. These three aspects are part of what Rubin has called the sex/gender system.[3] This concept, enunciated a quarter of a century ago, seems particularly appropriate to the understanding of Samoan masculinity with its subtle interplay of sex/gender. But contrary to Rubin, rather than biology being a fact of nature, a coat rack on which cultural constructions are thrown, here we are attempting to imagine it as a variable cultural category:

> a culturally specific set of ideas that might or might not be translatable into somewhat related ideas in other societies, but even when translatable could not be assumed to shape in cross-culturally similar ways each society's understanding of the male/female distinction.[4]

The sex/gender concept has made something of a theoretical comeback recently,[5] because it is especially helpful in those cultural contexts where there is a complex intertwining of what we might think of separately as sex, sexuality and gender. This is the case in Samoan thought, as explained both by our research participants, and by decades of scholarly work on the topic.

In the Samoan context, masculinity relates not just to sex and gender but also to kinship. There is little dispute that the sister–brother relationship is the pivotal one for Samoan society and culture.[6] This gendered kinship status does not map on to men and women; both men and women have secular and sacred statuses and male and female aspects. As a sister, the status of a female is sacred in relation to her brother. As a wife, a female's status is secular in relation to the sacred status of her husband's descent group.[7] The cross-sibling relationship is a template for others. Power, for example, has both female and male aspects, *mana* and *pule,* which can also be glossed as sacred/supernatural and secular.

In the brother–sister relationship, the sister is of higher status than her brother. The brother is responsible for, and is charged with the protection and control of his sister, especially of her purity. A brother must avoid any reference to his sister's sexuality. It is not that he is polluted by it. Rather, Schoeffel suggests, it is almost that she might be polluted by him: he must avoid his sister and her personal things, such as her sleeping mat, for fear of supernatural consequences.[8] Any attempt to dishonour her is an insult and an affront to him and their family. In an ideal world, this control and responsibility would be passed to the husband, and his family, at marriage.

Girls' sexuality is controlled by their brothers and other family members. This is a valued example of *amio* (individual impulses) being transformed into *aga (*socially controlled aspects of behaviour). Great attention is given to female sexuality and a major and definite social distinction is made between sisters and wives, girls and women in village life. But when it comes to the performance of gender, the code of dress and comportment, girls are allowed a little more laxity without being harshly ridiculed, as long as this behaviour is unable to be construed as sexual. In contrast, there is a relative unconcern about male sexuality, and the status or organisational distinction between husbands and brothers is relatively unmarked. Male sexual activity is a sign of *avi*, or virility, and males are not guarded as girls are. However, there is little leeway in male gendered behaviour. This is policed by accusations of being or becoming *fa'fafine* (the third gender of 'men acting as women'), which is strongly resisted by men who do not wish to be so classified. By establishing distance from *fa'afafine*, as well as by engaging in sexual activities with girls and/or women, boys demonstrate their masculinity. On the other hand, once established into the identity, a *fa'afafine* may choose to, and be permitted to, join in with the activities of the girls (*teine*) without posing any sexual threat to them.[9] Sexual maturity and sexual intercourse (sexuality) does not transform a boy into a man. Rather, it is the adult gender role of economic provision, particularly through establishing a marital-like relationship and supporting one's partner and children, that is the sign of male adulthood. In contrast, a girl (*teine*) becomes a woman (*fafine*) through the act of sexual intercourse.[10]

The sister–brother relationship has undergone considerable transformation and erosion in modernity while the formal attention given to the husband–wife relationship has grown, in accordance with *palagi* (white people's) customs in which the husband–wife relationship is the model for gender relations.[11] In the *palagi* model, particularly as introduced through Christian missions, the husband had the superior status. Hence the sacred bond, *feagaiga,* between brother and sister, which acted as the pre-eminent model of gender relations, has come to be rivalled by the husband–wife model. In the brother–sister model, the expression of sexuality is proscribed and the sister has the primary status; in the husband–wife model, sexuality is prescribed and the wife's status is secondary to her husband's.

Samoan people in Auckland

The Samoan reproduction study, on which this chapter is based, investigated the contexts and bases of decision-making about reproduction for some Samoan men and women in Auckland.[12] The fieldwork for the research took place between late 1997 and 1999.

Samoans in Auckland are part of a growing community whose origins are usually traced to the wave of migration from the Pacific Islands after the Second World War. At that time large numbers of Pacific peoples settled in New Zealand, especially in the cities of Auckland and Wellington, attracted by jobs in the growing economy, education, health care and new experiences. In 1962 a quota system for Western Samoans was introduced and subjected to variation over thc years, until in 1982 its legality was cast in doubt by a Privy Council ruling.[13] Under subsequent legislation, all Western Samoans present in New Zealand at that time were granted citizenship and future permanent residents qualified for citizenship. Like other Pacific peoples, Samoans (the 'Western' was dropped in 1999), were subjected to harassment during the various 'overstayers' campaigns, most notably in the later 1970s. Measures of income, home ownership, education and health indicate that Samoans, in common with other Pacific peoples, are disadvantaged in various ways in New Zealand, and in terms of income and employment, have lost ground with the economic downturn. However, in terms of political representation, recognition in the arts and sports, success in education and increase in life expectancy there are small but noticeable gains.

Typically, immigrants and descendants of Samoan immigrants maintain ties with their home islands and relatives who have migrated elsewhere, such as Australia or the US. Family-sponsored chain migration is common, as are visits in both directions and financial contributions to home affairs. Churches were, and are, a key cultural institution in *Niu Sila,* with around 92 per cent of

Samoans declaring a religious affiliation in 1996. Of all the Pacific groups in New Zealand, Samoans have the highest reported 'mother tongue' language ability, with nearly 70 per cent declaring competence in the Samoan language.[14]

Many migrants were integrated into the New Zealand labour force as semi-skilled workers in manufacturing, labouring, cleaning, the clothing industry, clerical work and care giving. Island-gained professional qualifications were frequently not recognised. With the downturn of the New Zealand economy in the mid-1970s and rapid technological change, this section of the working class bore disproportionate costs of the resultant restructuring, and later were adversely affected by the contracting of the welfare state. Although Pacific people in Aotearoa are predominantly still working class, many have also achieved educational success and occupational advancement to the point where there is a small but significant middle class.[15] Approximately three per cent of tertiary graduates each year are Pacific people, especially New Zealand-born ones.

Samoans comprise half the Pacific population in New Zealand, which now totals around 227,000, or six per cent, of the national population.[16] About two-thirds live in the Auckland area where they constitute approximately 11 per cent of the population.[17] This population is youthful, compared with the New Zealand population in general, and is growing faster than either the Maori or Pakeha segments. Both immigration and natural increase contributed to the Samoan population growth of 5.3 per cent (on average) between 1985 and 1991.[18] According to the 1996 census, over 90 per cent of Pacific youth in New Zealand are New Zealand-born.[19]

Our study

The study design included focused life-story interviews with eighty Samoan adults divided into four categories of twenty based on age (under or over forty years) and gender. Each group was interviewed by a researcher matched according to ethnicity, age and gender. Participants were members of the researchers' extensive social networks in Auckland Samoan communities, and were personally invited to participate. A sampling strategy to result in a cross-section of the community, based on church affiliation, place of residence and occupation, was employed.[20] It is not possible to make quantitative generalisations from this study. However, because of the multiple qualitative methods employed, which included the life-story interviews, focus groups and key person interviews, and the extensive community consultation undertaken when the report was drafted, the qualitative data are robust.

In comparing the two age groups of research participants we are also comparing a generation of Samoan men who were almost exclusively born and raised in Samoa (nineteen out of twenty), with a generation in which only one-fifth (four out of twenty) were born and raised in Samoa, an outcome of migration history. The older men's interviews were almost exclusively in the Samoan language, while the younger people's ones were largely in English.

Towards the end of the study, three men's focus groups were held, two with younger men, and one with the older group. Two women's focus groups were also held. The point of these groups was to get new information and feedback on themes that had been developed from the analysis of the interviews. These themes ranged through the value of children and parenthood, knowledge and practice of contraception, educational philosophy, the role of the churches in sexuality and relationship education, notions of courtship and related themes. Finally, about twenty key person interviews were conducted to incorporate the perspectives of community workers and health professionals, officials from government ministries, ministers of religion, and community leaders. The key persons were identified on the basis of the researchers' knowledge and the advice of our Samoan advisory group.

Our research was focused on those aspects of sex and gender that relate to reproduction, because it was aimed at answering some questions about family planning, contraception, sexuality, parenthood and related areas, as specified in our Health Research Council of New Zealand research grant. Although we had intended to include *fa'afafine,* none volunteered for the study. We also hoped to include some homosexual men and women but everyone who participated identified as heterosexual. Thus our findings relate only to the experiences of men and women who identify as heterosexual and of masculine or feminine gender.

Men's perceptions and experiences of sex and gender

Older men

When they were young men growing up in Samoa, the older participants did hard physical work, and were under sometimes harsh parental discipline, but they were not under close surveillance like the girls. Although parents and other senior relatives might encourage the boys to refrain from sexual activity, there was also encouragement from peers and more general tacit expectation that boys would 'experiment'.

From the perspectives of these older men, the development of interest in the opposite sex was an inevitable corollary of human development, a natural fact, expressed in the terms of popular conceptions of the western sciences of biology or chemistry in phrases such as, 'cells matured', or 'chemistry between their body cells'. During adolescence and later, having sex with lots of women was seen as natural, 'the way of men', and it was something over which men had no control because it was a biological urge.

ae pei ona ou ta'ua i le amataga, o lagona o le soifuaga e le mafai one 'aveesea, o le natura o le tagata, e iai ona lagona i tulaga fa'apea, i le age ua tatau ona fai lagona ia

Having lots of sex was a sign of vitality – *avi* – and masculinity. Consequently, a number of men had several children outside of their marriage or de facto relationships both before and while they were 'married'.

In certain situations, for example when repeated pregnancies endangered one's partner's health, or with repeated infidelities, having lots of sex was negatively evaluated in a rather mild way, e.g. as a 'weakness'. A husband who was 'playing around' while his wife was pregnant was also thought to risk endangering the health of the foetus or newborn. But, these instances aside, in general an active sex life was valued. Two of the older men who had been widowed recommended that men in their situation should marry younger women to keep their vitality.

The fathers of men in this age group did not talk to their unmarried sons about sex, nor did the sons ask. In many cases, the fathers knew about their sons' sexual exploits but would not discuss them directly. For the sons to ask questions would be cheeky and presumptuous *(tautalaitiiti)* as they were not at the stage where such information was appropriate. That stage would occur only when they settled down with a partner and had children. Rather, as adolescents, they picked up information mainly from eaves-dropping on the conversations of somewhat older boys, especially their relations – a method also reported by Schoeffel.[21] Boys would never talk with their sisters about such things because of the relationship of respect between sisters and brothers.

Courtship could be open *(fa'amalamalamaga)* only where there was a clear intention of marriage. Otherwise it was hidden *(fa'apouliuli)* at least until the young couple was discovered or the woman became obviously pregnant. At this time their relationship might be publicly recognised, which might entail getting married. The polite terms for sexual relations were framed only in terms of 'making families'. The idea of openly dating a series of young women simply did not arise. Equally unknown was the concept of a platonic relationship of friendship with a woman. A relationship or encounter between young people of the opposite sex would inevitably be framed as sexual. Thus if a girl put herself outside the protection of her family, and especially of her brothers, by going out by herself at night, or going to a remote corner of the island, a boy would construe this as tacit consent to a sexual relationship. Such encounters and hidden relationships often led to marriage or settled relationships. This understanding of sexual risk was common to both the older men and women in this study. The women agreed that under these circumstances it was almost impossible to say 'No' to sexual advances. One man discussed the practice of *toso teine*, or 'pulling girls for sex', in such circumstances, as something which was now frowned upon especially because of its resemblance to the Western concept of rape. He stated that he himself had felt no need to indulge in this practice because he was very attractive to women!

Some of the older men were very forthright in their views that young men were only after one thing: sex, and they advised their daughters accordingly, while cautioning their sons and other young men in their care, to respect their girlfriends and not to expect to have sex with them the first time they went out together. In this way they were simultaneously conveying the ideas about opposite-sex relationships that they had grown up with, while trying to counter these ideas in the younger generation.

The older men did not discuss *moetotolo* or 'night crawling',[22] but this was an issue for their female contemporaries in the study. Even when they were well within the protection of their own families, young women might be sexually violated by young men, who were out to demonstrate their bravery and *avi,* or perhaps had revenge in mind, creeping into their *fale* at night. As Tcherkézoff explains, *moetotolo* is not equivalent to the French or English usages of 'viol' or 'rape', as, by definition, it takes place only when the girl is under the protection of her family, and it does not usually involve intercourse. This practice needs to be understood within its cultural context which includes, at the most elementary level, traditional Samoan nuptial practices, concepts of day and night on one hand, and night and day on the other, and notions of the family control and value of female sexuality.

The statements of the older participants supported the ethnographic literature in that while sexual activity was a valued part of being a male, it was not the sole measure of adult Samoan masculinity. Economic provision for the family and to meet other church and community obligations was the prime feature of adult male responsibility. It was pre-eminent over, for example, sexual fidelity within marriage or the sharing of childcare and other household responsibilities. Taking on economic responsibility was a hallmark of 'settling down to have children'. A few of the older men spoke about how consideration for one's wife and children was an important part of the husband and father's role, but everyone (i.e., the older men and older women) agreed that economic provision was the major contribution for men.

Men wanted to become fathers to have children to love, care for and instruct; to have another generation to carry on the genealogy *(gafa)* or family name (especially important for sons); and to have someone to care for them in their old age and to contribute to the family work and finances. Children were universally seen as God's blessings, and women as particularly designed to be mothers and to care for children. Wives and mothers, not husbands and fathers, were seen as those who should be responsible for preventing pregnancy, if this were necessary. However, there were few recognised reasons for preventing pregnancy according to the men in this age group. Chief among them was their partner's health. The availability of resources to care for the children was noted by some men as a consideration which was becoming increasingly important for the next generation of parents, especially in New Zealand, where the care and education of children was more costly than in Samoa. However, the older male participants themselves rarely questioned their own ability to provide resources for their families, so closely was this connected to their sense of adulthood. Nonetheless, one of the older men confessed that he had apologised to his family for not always being able to provide for them, despite his best efforts. The responsibility of a father to provide for his children was often expressed in terms of not only providing 'enough to eat' but also in providing clothes and schooling and, more generally, in providing childhoods free from hardship, and giving their children guidance or discipline. There was acknowledgement that these ideals were not always achieved. A few of the men mentioned that despite the idea that children were blessings, child abuse was a problem in the Samoan community, and one which should be openly acknowledged.

After living many years in New Zealand and adapting to a situation where both partners often had paid jobs, a few of the men were adept at doing household chores which were strictly women's work in Samoa, such as doing the family laundry. Several of the older men and women recounted humorous episodes about relations visiting from Samoa, who when they observed the men doing the wash, took great exception. One visiting relative actually moved out of the household to live with other family members with more acceptable gendered behaviour, while others made comments which showed their disgust. This demonstrates the relative importance that clearly defined gender roles have in Samoan definitions of masculinity for men in this age group, and the tendency of some men in New Zealand, especially the younger ones, to exhibit more flexibility.

Summary of sex and gender in the older men's narratives of experience

In general, Shore's model, with its emphasis on gender rather than sexuality, sums up the older men's experience and perceptions rather well, although the real-life situations are, of course, rather more varied than the model suggests. It is economic provision in a settled relationship which determines their status as adult men, not their sexual exploits; in other words, masculine gender, not masculine sexuality, is what 'makes a man'. That the only mention of *fa'afafine* in the older men's narratives served to distance themselves from this gender category lends further support to Shore's contention that it is gendered behaviour rather than sexuality which comes in for greater attention in the achievement of respected masculinity.

Younger men

Although there are some strong continuities between the older men and younger men in terms of perceptions and experiences, there are also clear differences. More of the younger men had had discussions with their parents about sexuality and relationships. For most, however, such topics were out of bounds. They would be told off, just as the older men had once been, if they were so bold as to ask questions. From this they learned that sex or talking about it, or both, were bad. Several reported being made to cover their eyes if any form of sexual intimacy came on the television. At church they learned that brothers and sisters should not talk about sexual things. At school, many of them were exposed to sex education classes, which they found particularly embarrassing. They did not observe their parents being affectionate to each other and thus learned that open display of affection between partners was not seemly. However, one or two noted that they knew their parents loved each other because of how they helped each other.

Like the older generation, they got information about sex through older male relatives, as well as through the media. They, too, explained their sexual liaisons in terms of biology and chemistry: that it was in the nature of men and was something that they could do little about. Younger men were able, in English, to discuss casual dating and the possibility of friendships with girls. They were also able to discuss sexual relationships separately from the concept of forming families. While being able to discuss these matters in English was part of the reason for this generational change, perhaps as important was seeing that such relationships were possible in the lives of friends and acquaintances. This created quite a different context from that of their older counterparts for understanding relationships with the opposite sex.

Several of the younger men expressed quite ambivalent attitudes towards women. This was manifest in their discussions of feeling fearful of relationships, disregarding women's safety or feelings while at the same time expressing positive interest in forming relationships with women. Alcohol was seen as a means of getting up courage to approach a girl, a function also noted by the older men. Consequently, quite a few first sexual encounters were undertaken in a drunken state without either partner using contraception. However, as a group, compared with the older men, there was not the same emphasis on having many sexual partners. Like the older men, the younger men did not show any deviation from an assumption of heterosexuality, and mentioned *fa'afafine* only in order to demonstrate rejection:

> I was about thirteen or fourteen and I was asleep at a friend's place. A *fa'afafine* tried to fondle me and that was quite freaky. I turned around and punched him in the mouth. I was a friend of his brother.

When the younger men talked about growing up and becoming adults most of them did so only in relation to marital-type relationships. However a few discussed other adult gender roles: for example, being the main breadwinner for the family including parents and younger siblings, or, being very protective of your sisters as a young adult, because by then you know 'what guys are like, and they are creeps'. Thus the husband-wife relationship dominated the young men's models of gender relationships.

Younger men did not discuss the practice of *toso teine* or *moetotolo* and although one young man described a situation where he had forced himself on his sexual partner, he was well aware of the Western construction of rape which would be put on this situation. Young women noted that men in this age group who were recent arrivals from Samoa did not seem to understand the concept of 'no', in contrast to New Zealand-raised boys who were much less 'forward'. As well as confirming changes in notions of sexuality, the women's observation also shows that what we are constructing as a generational change within New Zealand is not necessarily able to be extrapolated back to Samoa. Indeed it might be interpreted as both a generational change and a change between Samoans in Samoa and Samoans in New Zealand.

In relation to their gender and kinship roles as husbands and fathers, the younger men, like their older counterparts, stressed the economic role of provider as their primary role: 'As a Samoan man, basically, it's always just to provide, you know. You're the number one.' However, they were much more likely than the older men to add other responsibilities such as caring for the children, doing household chores, or caring for their wives. More younger men were prepared to do chores, like laundry, and to share decisions, recognising that this was a major change from their fathers' generation: 'All the decisions have to be done together, not like the Samoans have often done – having the man decide everything.'

A large proportion believed that contraception was a shared responsibility. Like the older men, quite a few had had a number of different sexual relationships which they referred to quite freely. None of these, however, was an extramarital relationship. In addition, half of this younger group thought that premarital chastity for men was desirable. Sometimes this was based on hindsight gained from their own experience of several sexual relationships before they had 'settled down'. Compared with the older men, 'settled relationships' for these younger men were much more likely to include not only economic provision but also an idea of sexual fidelity. This was a clear and important difference between the two age groups.Like the older men, the younger men thought of children as God's blessings who should be accepted. However, more men in this group were inclined to stress that to look after these growing blessings required more economic resources in New Zealand. Consequently, families needed to be spaced and limited in size, so that the children could be looked after properly. Discussion about the limits to their ability to provide for a large number of children did not appear to run the risk of diminishing their masculine status in the way it would have done for some of the older men. Many also acknowledged that both partners contributed to the family economic resources, even if men were still thought to be the main provider.

Carrying on the *fa'a Samoa* (the Samoan way) was an important theme in the context of bringing up their children properly for both generations, in terms of instilling in the children a sense of family obligations and values. Although he did not refer directly to the *feagaiga,* one younger father described how in his two-storeyed house the girls were upstairs and the boys were downstairs and when the cousins or other visitors came over, they were always expected to socialise in the public rooms, not the bedrooms. This spatial arrangement assisted the continuation of a respect relationship between his sons and daughters. Another noted that if he went into his sister's room, he was to sit on the floor. Some younger men thought the *feagaiga* was only relevant in Samoa.

These younger men were quite determined that part of their role as fathers was to provide their children with values and knowledge so that information and advice about sexuality, relationships and marriage could be shared. In this regard the younger men were deviating from the older Samoan educational practice where a person had to be at the appropriate stage before the information relating to that stage was imparted. These younger men hoped that they could prepare their children for the stage ahead.

Summary – sex and gender in the younger men's narratives

For the younger men, some aspects of Shore's model are no longer applicable, although this is a matter of degree. It is possible to argue that for the younger men there is a greater convergence of sex/gender and that the achievement of a respected adult masculinity requires attention both to sexuality and to gender performance. Despite the continued distancing from *fa'afafine*, men may carry out chores that were formerly designated as women's work without being subjected to the caustic comment that the older generation would have encountered. While the younger men's primary role is still seen by both genders as economic provision for the family, this role has been expanded to include household chores and childcare. There is some recognition that there may be limits to economic provision by the husband/father in the current New Zealand context. There is a greater emphasis on sexual fidelity for men in their role as husbands, some suggestion that men should exercise sexual restraint before marriage, and a much greater acceptance of shared responsibility and control between husband and wife over the number and spacing of their children.

Discussion

Shore's model is useful in this discussion of generational change because it allows for systematic consideration of local models of sex and gender. Among the other changes going on in the sex and gender order is an increasing flexibility in gender performance for the younger heterosexual men, accompanied by a greater attention to and an increased social constraint on heterosexual expression. In Shore's terms, male sexuality and gender both come in for attention in the younger ages.

In both age groups sexuality is discussed in terms of biology, and a rather deterministic biology at that. This research did not explore these biological images in detail but they appear to be not too dissimilar to popular Western scientific notions of hormonal changes, body chemistry 'urges' and related notions that saturate the popular media.[23]

The emphasis on economic provision as a key role for adult men has remained relatively constant, despite employment difficulties for many Samoan men in New Zealand, although other responsibilities have been added to adult masculinity for those who live in this country. Indeed, many men now see the importance of being able to provide adequately for one's children as a key factor, and along with the health of the mother and children, is a reason for limiting family size or spacing the births of children, and may be argued as a father's Christian duty to his children. This viewpoint is, however, sometimes in contestation with the idea, more common in the older generation, that children are God's blessings and should be accepted as such.

Glossary of Samoan Terms

Aga	socially controlled aspects of behaviour
Amio	individual impulses
Avi	one who has sexual prowess
Fa'afafine	a man who acts as a woman
Fa'amalamalamaga	to make clear, explain; the practice of public courtship
Fa'apouliuli	to shut out, darken,
Fa'aSamoa	the Samoan way
Fafine	woman
Fale	house
Feagaiga	a covenant, especially between brother and sister
Gafa	one's family, lineage, genealogy
Mana	an aspect of power
Moetotolo	night creeping
Palagi	European
Pule	an aspect of power
Teine	girl
Toso teine	'pulling' girls

The authors acknowledge the generosity of all participants, the input of the Advisory Group and staff of the Pacific Health Research Centre, and the support of their respective departments at the University of Auckland. The study was funded by the Health Research Council of New Zealand. Julie Park also acknowledges visiting fellowships at the Australian National University, Canberra, in 1999 at the National Centre for Epidemiology and Population Health and the Gender Relations Project.

three

Living the contradictions: A Foucauldian examination of my youthful rugby experiences

RICHARD PRINGLE

> Rugby is impossible to escape, and it's heading in a direction which is increasingly harmful to New Zealand, and men in particular.[1]

> From the time I saw the All Blacks run on to the park that first time, like a spill of black opals on green baize, I was hooked for life. They have never let me down. They have lost the occasional match, but it has never been because they gave up or because they did not play their hearts out to the last seconds. Because they have the guts to win, even when perhaps they should in theory lose, they represent, to me anyway, the best characteristics of the New Zealand male: resilience, courage, toughness, enterprise, innovation and perseverance.[2]

In Aotearoa New Zealand rugby union is often experienced and made sense of in intensely different ways. Rugby has been variously defined as a sport for gentlemen or barbarians,[3] as an élitist or egalitarian sport,[4] and even as a way of life or secular religion;[5] but more typically as a *man's* sport and rarely, if ever, a woman's. Critical social commentators have labelled rugby as a producer and supporter of masculine hegemony,[6] and succinctly as violent:[7] 'Other sports may become violent but rugby *is* violent – remove the violence and you no longer have the game.'[8] In brief, New Zealand writers tend to either celebrate or critique the notion that rugby is 'our national game'.[9]

Whether we 'love it, hate it or try to be indifferent to it, rugby union football shapes New Zealand social history and everyday life'.[10] Hence, critical examination of the social influence of rugby in Aotearoa is an important topic. In particular, given the highly aggressive nature of rugby and its close connections with nationalism and men, I am concerned with how rugby helps shape male subjectivities and relations of power.

In this chapter, to help gain an understanding of rugby's influence in the construction of masculinities, I use the ideas of Michel Foucault to examine my youthful experiences in rugby. More specifically, I examine how dominating discourses associated with rugby – being male, and being a respectful person –

have interacted in a complex and at times contradictory manner in helping to shape my sense of self. Although the concept of hegemonic masculinity currently provides a dominant framework for analysing sport and masculinities, I aim to promote Foucauldian ideas as useful for understanding the complexities, contradictions and fragmentations of the male sporting self. Finally, by revealing my personal struggle with rugby, I hope to contribute to the challenge of the prominent place of rugby in New Zealand culture.

I begin this chapter by providing an overview of the social influence of rugby in New Zealand, followed by an introduction to the ideas of Foucault. I finish by telling my story of rugby experiences, interweaving it with Foucauldian insights.

A DISCURSIVE EXAMINATION OF RUGBY IN AOTEAROA NEW ZEALAND

Social constructionists typically portray sport as a leading definer of masculinity that helps link males and produce male dominance in society.[11] Indeed, the very visible performance of moving bodies in sports settings, coupled with the arguably excessive amount of attention New Zealand culture gives to sport, help make sport a 'crucial arena of struggle over basic social conceptions of masculinity and femininity'.[12] Within Aotearoa the prime sport that has helped shape masculinities and gender relations is rugby union.

Since the early 1900s rugby has been typically viewed as ideal for instilling manly character in boys, developing their physical strength and 'providing a suitable channel for (male) adolescent energies'.[13] These beliefs were, in part, inherited through the colonisation process but were also politically promoted.[14] For example, the success of the tour of England and Wales by the 1905 New Zealand men's rugby team (nicknamed the All Blacks during this tour) was strategically seized upon by politicians to help forge a national identity. Phillips asserts that at the beginning of the twentieth century New Zealanders were suffering something of a national identity crisis: Pakeha predominantly viewed New Zealand as a small outpost of the English 'motherland' and tensions between Maori and Pakeha were extreme.[15] Therefore, the victories of the 1905 All Blacks, when Britain was a dominant world power, provided political fodder that Premier Richard Seddon used to laud the benefits of the 'healthy' New Zealand lifestyle and the 'egalitarian' and 'unifying' nature of rugby. Rugby was soon deemed in the media as 'our national game' and as a panacea for fears that urban males were becoming effeminate.[16] A dominating discourse soon developed that promoted rugby as a maker of tough New Zealand men.

Even today, dominating discourses in New Zealand construct rugby as a '*real* man's game' and as 'our national game'. These discourses act to position rugby as a positive social force that helps unite New Zealand through providing a national identity. This quixotic set of beliefs in part reflects the historical dominance of men in New Zealand society, and that 'until the early 1970s the game was culturally central, compulsory for schoolboys, popular and an inescapable feature of life in New Zealand's small-scale communities'.[17] At the same time, these rugby discourses problematically position females and males who are not closely involved in rugby as unimportant in New Zealand social life.

A recent interview study of eighty New Zealand males with haemophilia helps reveal an adverse influence of these problematic rugby discourses. Park concludes although the health risk from haemophilia is serious, even life-threatening in some cases, the inability to play rugby is 'the single most pervasive idiom of distress for men with haemophilia'.[18] One teenage boy who suffered from the invisible disease of haemophilia, for example, stated 'I'd rather have my legs cut off so people could see it.'[19] Such is the impact of the omnipresent disciplinary effect of a discourse that suggests if you are a New Zealand boy and do not play rugby, you are not normal.

Furthermore, the dominating discourses that surround rugby are problematic in another way. They promote the celebration of a sport that encourages the use of aggression, physical intimidation and acts of violence. Although many New Zealanders would think of rugby as a hard and aggressive sport, with a relatively high chance that its participants will sustain some degree of physical injury, perhaps few would label rugby as violent. The word 'violent' is often used in conjunction with illegal acts of physical aggression designed to inflict pain. Violence is therefore an emotive concept commonly associated with criminal or deviant behaviour and not with 'our national' sport. However, Coakley reports that in heavy contact sports, such as rugby, 'intimidation and violence have become widely used as strategies for winning games, promoting individual careers, and increasing profits for sponsors'.[20]

Winning in rugby is undoubtedly reliant on the use of physical force, acts of physical aggression and ability to withstand pain. In this sense, the rugby body becomes normalised as a physical weapon.[21] The more ably a rugby participant can run over or through other players, or knock them to the ground in 'crunching' tackles or 'big hits', the more respected that player becomes. Furthermore, illegal play involving punching or other deliberate pain-inflicting techniques – which are generally euphemised as over-vigorous play, retaliation or niggle – is often accepted as legitimate play in particular contexts.[22] Although few rugby participants would say they play rugby to deliberately hurt players, many may admit they play 'hard' in order to dominate the opposition in an attempt to win.

A result of this 'competitive' attitude is many rugby players eventually suffer from injuries, and the New Zealand taxpayer is left with a large financial cost. In the 1997/98 financial year, new and ongoing rugby injury claims rose to over $25 million.[23] Most of this sum was for male players aged between fifteen and thirty-four years. And the reported cause of injury for over fifty per cent of these claims involved being struck by another person, collision, or being knocked over. Two of the injury claims were for actual deaths on the rugby field.[24] In total, the financial cost to the New Zealand tax player for rugby injuries equates to over $184 dollars per year for each adult rugby participant. However, the cost of rugby's sporting dominance in New Zealand is more than just financial. In particular, repeated concern has been expressed about rugby's relationship with violence, both on and off the field, and masculinities.[25]

Violence, in its various forms, is often recognised as one of the major social problems of our times.[26] Although many people may view violence as a breakdown of normal social behaviours, it can also be viewed as part of 'what we are, an expression of deep and extensive cultural patterns'.[27] In this sense, I am concerned about the connections between men and violence. New Zealand statistics, for example, overwhelmingly indicate that men are both the victims and perpetrators of most violence.[28] The strong connection between males and violence has lead Kenway and Fitzclarence to argue that violence can be understood as an expression of a particular type of masculinity, and that particular sports, such as rugby, are implicated in the construction of these masculinities. They state:

> Male dominance/subordination relations are often worked out through legitimate (sport) and illegitimate (brawling, bashing) physical violence. Again, such violence is premised on beliefs about the importance of aggressive and violent acts for gaining and maintaining status, reputation and resources in the male group, to sustain a sense of masculine identity and as a form of 'self' protection.[29]

Reports of sports stars and their off-field acts of violence, such as O.J. Simpson and Mike Tyson, often gain headline news. Similarly, the off-field violence of professional rugby player Romi Ropati gained media attention in Aotearoa New Zealand. In 1999, Ropati pleaded guilty to assaulting Peter Attwood in central Dunedin. The vicious attack happened several hours after his team, the Otago Highlanders, were beaten in the Super 12 rugby final. Attwood suffered two fractures to his jaw requiring reconstructive surgery. Two of his teeth were broken and had to be removed, and he had facial bruising and swelling. The prime explanation for Ropati's violence revolved around his disappointment in losing the rugby. This is the second serious assault charge Ropati has faced, yet his criminal record of violence has not adversely affected his professional rugby career.

The connection between the violent behaviour of men in sporting contexts and violent behaviour outside sport is often speculated about. However, it is only relatively recently that research has begun to closely examine the assumed connections. A survey of North American university sportsmen found that a belief in the value of toughness in sport is related to aggressive acts off the sports field.[30] Similarly, a study of reported sexual assaults at American universities reveals that male student-athletes, when compared to the rest of the male student population, are involved in a significantly higher percentage of assaults.[31] In New Zealand, Ritchie reports that men who have played rugby as adults are more likely to endorse the use of violence in various social situations, in comparison to men who have not played rugby.[32]

However, given the complexity of human behaviours, these quantitative studies cannot conclude that participation in violent sports actually causes males to be violent off the field. It is possible, for example, that those who choose to play rugby are already more likely to view violence as socially appropriate in certain situations. Nevertheless, these studies help legitimate concerns about the relationship between the violence celebrated in rugby and violence off the field. They also help indicate that we should be concerned with, or at least need to further examine, the social influence of rugby in New Zealand.

The complexity of understanding rugby's impact on masculinities

Attempting to understand how rugby impacts on male subjectivities is complex. Nevertheless, I am concerned that the prevalence of rugby in New Zealand helps link and glorify an influential way of being male with sporting prowess, acceptance of some acts of violence, and tolerance of pain. In other words, rugby helps produce a dominating discourse of masculinity which informs that 'real men' are tough, aggressive, physically superior to others, risk-takers, and competitive. The dominance of this discourse, therefore, acts to marginalise other more gentle and respectful ways of being male. However, it would be erroneous to believe this dominating discourse of masculinity exclusively produces New Zealand men who are consistently unreflective and uncritical about violence, pain and relations of power.

New Zealand males are clearly influenced by a range of discourses and bodily experiences which impact on their subjectivities. For example, young males are often encouraged in various contexts to be respectful of others, and increasingly men are disciplined to take care of their bodies through various practices, such as moderation in alcohol consumption, safe sex and safe driving practices. Furthermore, the second wave of feminism and the gay rights movement have also impacted strongly on understandings of masculinities and femininities. New Zealand men, under the postmodern condition,[33] are therefore influenced by multiple and competing discourses which come to the fore in a pastiche of different social contexts. Hence, gaining a clear understanding of acceptable ways of being male, and a coherent sense of self, can be a complex and difficult process for many males.

This negotiation of manliness is further complicated by the reality that rugby culture is not one-dimensional, but is also constituted through multiple and, at times, contradictory discourses. Rugby, for example, although often violent can also promote 'fair and gentlemanly' play, where written and unwritten rules and codes of honour are closely adhered to. And importantly, primarily since 1981 a more openly critical view of rugby and its associated practices have developed. The hard man image of a player who can take a 'few knocks' and 'dish out punishment' is now more likely to draw public criticism. For example, Phillips asserts the infamous 1992 eye-gouging incident performed by ex-All Black Richard Loe on Greg Cooper made him better known as a folk-devil than a hero,[34] and less vicious practices have been widely frowned on.

The explicit commodification of rugby has also impacted on images of masculinity.[35] The All Blacks are no longer solely depicted as narrow caricatures of traditional masculinity; they can now commonly be viewed in glossy magazines as caring partners, in self-effacing television commercials, or even as the hosts of documentaries on being good fathers. All of these contribute to a softer and rounder image of masculinity, in contrast to the image of dominant masculinity that is glorified on the field. Hence, New Zealand men may not only experience rugby in very different ways, but individuals may also have difficulty in developing a coherent understanding of rugby.

Recognising the complexity of social forces that interplay in the construction of fluid masculine subjectivities, Whannel argues 'there is a pressing need to understand masculinities in the round – as dominant but also contradictory; contradictory, but also dominant'.[36] He also stresses the need to understand how 'sport has the appearance of being that which unites men; yet it is also a practice that divides men'.[37] With these concerns in mind, I have turned to the work of Michel Foucault to help us understand the influence of rugby in the construction of fragmented masculine subjectivities.

A growing number of feminists have used poststructuralism, particularly the work of Foucault, to help understand the complexities of subjectivities and the dynamics of gender relations.[38] Star, for example, boldly argues that Foucauldian accounts of the connections between discourse, power and subjectivity have been responsible for revitalising theorising about masculinities.[39] In the following section, I introduce and promote select aspects of Foucauldian thought.

Introducing Foucauldian ideas

Foucault summarises his overall scholarly focus by stating 'my objective for more than twenty-five years has been to sketch out a history of the different ways in our culture that humans develop knowledge about themselves'.[40] In essence, Foucault's work is concerned with how the workings of discourse and power constitute subjects or individuals.

Foucault considers that discourses should be treated as 'practices that systematically form the objects of which they speak'.[41] Discourse, therefore, structures our way of thinking, forms social relations, and constructs our subjectivities. Hence, the discourses available to people in particular social contexts discursively locate or position them. In this sense, discourse creates subject positions from which people can exercise varying social influence or power; 'it is in discourse that power and knowledge are joined together'.[42] Given there are multiple and competing discourses, Foucault asserts that the subject positions created are never stable.[43] People, therefore, will at times have to negotiate the associated inner tensions of competing discourses.

Foucault does not view individuals deterministically as discursive dupes. In contrast, he aims to show that people 'are much freer than they feel, that people accept as truth, as evidence, some themes which have built up at a certain moment during history, and this so-called evidence can be criticised and destroyed'.[44] Hence, his notion of the constructed self clearly allows for a type of agency; although individuals are constituted by discourse, they are still capable of critically reflecting on how certain discourses have developed. Individuals can therefore act to change their subject positions or subjectivities through exercising 'some choice with respect to the discourses and practices' they use.[45]

Foucault asserts that social change can occur when marginalised and repressed discourses are revealed and these alternative ways of thinking, or cleavages of resistance, are opened up. Nevertheless, Foucault warns that we should not imagine a social world simplistically divided between accepted (dominant) and excluded discourse as there are a 'multiplicity of discursive elements that come into play in various strategies'.[46] Thus, we should not think that there is just one discourse that surrounds males and rugby; but multiple discourses that have varying, and at times contradictory, influence in differing social contexts.

Discourse and power can be viewed as productive as they constitute subjects, power relations and our social realities. Foucault rejects that power is primarily repressive in its exercise, as he doubts that people would continue to accept or obey a repressive or coercive form of power.[47] Consequently, he argues against the traditional model in which power is presented as 'possessed' by an élite class or by a certain group of people, and acts repressively in a top-down manner on those without power. Instead, he asserts that power is omnipresent, as it is produced through all actions and relations between people. 'Power is exercised from innumerable points, in the interplay of nonegalitarian and mobile relations.'[48] He does not deny the potential existence of global forms of domination, such as sexism, but believes that to understand the workings of globalised relations, one needs to conduct an ascending analysis of power. An ascending analysis examines how 'power relations at the micro-level of society make possible certain global effects of domination, such as class power and patriarchy'.[49]

In contrast, Connell's concepts of hegemonic masculinity and the gender order appear underpinned by a traditional view of power.[50] Although Connell would deny that power always acts repressively – as under hegemony theory power primarily operates via consent – he nevertheless argues that power is *held* by a dominant group of males, and it operates in a top-down manner on marginalised and subordinated males and, more generally, on females. For example, Connell and his colleagues assert that understanding how a particular definition of masculinity becomes hegemonic requires an examination of 'how particular groups of men inhabit positions of power and wealth and how they legitimate and reproduce the social relationships that generate their dominance'.[51] Connell's reliance on what Star calls the 'rather moribund "power-over/down" hegemony model',[52] has resulted in several recent critiques.[53] For example, Miller is critical of the grandness associated with the concept of hegemonic masculinity, as he asserts it attempts to explain 'everything and nothing in a circular motion, tending to lack a dynamic of history made at specific sites'.[54] Indeed, Connell's 'big picture' account of gender relations does not satisfactorily explain completely what he calls the 'anomalies' of the gender order, such as the successful gay businessman or the influential female politician. Furthermore, although his big-picture view of the gender order portrays masculinities as multiple, it also tends to portray male identities as stable, coherent and rational, thus glossing over the complexities and contradictions associated with notions of self.

In contrast, Foucault contends that each discourse has a specific history, and the power effects of each discourse remain influential through specific social mechanisms or tactics or complex strategies. Foucault, therefore, believes that our understandings of power and its impact on social interactions and behaviours should be studied through specific historical or genealogical analyses, not assumed from a general or grand theory of social processes.

Furthermore, Foucault contends that the intimate relationship between discourse and power is unstable, as discourse can similarly produce or reproduce power while also challenging and undermining its effect. In this sense discourse can be 'both an instrument and an effect of power, but also a hindrance, a stumbling-block, a point of resistance and a starting point for an opposing strategy'.[55] Foucault therefore highlights the notion that where there is power there is also resistance.

The 1981 South African Springbok tour of New Zealand and the subsequent large-scale protests provide a good example of this power resistance notion. For example, it is probable that rugby's influential social position within New Zealand, due to its being our national sport and thus symbolising the national identity, was partly responsible for why the tour drew so much protest.

I speculate that if it had been a South African women's water polo team that toured New Zealand in 1981, it would have generated much smaller protest, and probably not have culminated in aerial flour bag bombing of the swimming pool, as happened in the final test match of the rugby.

Subjectifying and objectifying people into docile bodies

Foucault's schema of three modes of objectification of the subject (scientific classification, dividing practices and subjectification) provides a useful framework for further introducing his ideas. Scientific classification, the first mode of objectification, is concerned primarily with how the human sciences construct influential discourses or knowledges so that people come to recognise themselves as both objects and subjects of knowledge.[56] The second mode of objectification is closely tied to the workings of science and has been called 'dividing practices'. Foucault explains the subject is both internally divided and divided from others. 'Essentially "dividing practices" are modes of manipulation that combine the mediation of a science (or pseudo-science) and the practice of exclusion – usually in a spatial sense, but always in a social one'.[57] Foucault asserts that scientific knowledge is used to justify divisions between the mad and sane, the sick and well, the gay and straight, and the deviant and normal.[58] And these knowledges, which are culturally and historically specific, can produce oppressive power relations. For example, the 'stigma attached to the mad, the sick, the criminal, the black, the poor, the unemployed, and so on, provides an objectification that not only classifies and contains the deviant but also "normalises" the rest of the population'.[59]

The concept of dividing practices was incorporated into Foucault's notion of 'technologies of power', which he defines as a technology which 'determine(s) the conduct of individuals and submit(s) them to certain ends or domination, an objectivizing of the subject'.[60] In this sense, Foucault regards dividing practices as a disciplinary technique. Foucault illustrates that disciplinary techniques, such as surveillance, normalisation, and rituals of exclusion, lead to the creation of the disciplinary society and the 'meticulous control of the operations of the body'.[61] Hence, the workings of an omnipresent and disciplinary power produce social bodies that are subject to a 'political anatomy of detail', and thus, bodies can be thought of as docile but productive.[62]

These first two modes of objectification – scientific classification and dividing practices – are considered by Foucault to represent just one side of the 'art of governing people', as these modes represent people as passively dominated or constrained.[63] In contrast, Foucault's third mode of objectification, 'subjectification', is concerned with techniques that people actively use to constitute and transform themselves – that is, 'techniques or practices of self'.

Foucault states that practices of self-formation can be thought of as an 'exercise of self upon self by which one tries to work out, to transform one's self and to attain a certain mode of being'.[64] In essence, Foucault asserts that people help constitute themselves as 'a work of art'.

However, Foucault asserts these practices of self are not something the individual invents, but are 'patterns that he *[sic]* finds in his culture and which are proposed, suggested and imposed on him by his culture, his society and his social group'.[65] Thus, although the rugby player with shaved head or nose studs and tattoos may think that he or she is a unique self-creation, these appearances can also be thought of as influenced by the workings of discourse. Likewise, Sparkes[66] cautiously reminds us that we do not have complete control over the meanings we make about ourselves. He reports the dominating discourses available in our culture, such as the ones related to age, gender, sexuality, health, ethnicity and beauty, influence who we think we are and who we think we can become. Dominating discourses can, therefore, act to privilege some people while disadvantaging others.

In the following section I use a Foucauldian perspective to examine how the workings of discourse associated with being a male rugby player provided me with specific advantages but also rigidly normalised my behaviours.

Reflections on my hypermasculine experiences in rugby

My youthful experiences in rugby provide the prime reason why I am currently undertaking research on the social influence of rugby, and why I am lecturing on sporting issues at a university. Rugby has not only helped shape my career but it has also helped shape how I view others and myself. Perhaps strangely, it was my earliest involvement in rugby which had the largest impact on me. In my last two years of primary school (aged nine to eleven years), I played in the red jersey of Stoke Tahunanui and was coached by my beloved teacher, Mrs Longly. And for two years straight we never lost a game. It was here that I began to think of myself as a rugged, fast and skilled rugby player; as one of the boys. This self-image became what Hall might describe as my 'comforting story of self'.[67] I relished the status I gained from my teachers and peers for my abilities to run with the ball and score tries. And at this age I never worried about getting hurt. We had not yet learnt that winning was more important than pain-free bodies, so the tackles were gentle and never a punch was thrown. Rugby, I believed, was a grand game.

Primary-school rugby was a prime dividing practice that distinguished between boys and girls, and between the boys. Girls were not allowed to play rugby, and this helped affirm my then 'essentialised understanding' that girls were physically weaker and less skilled. Rugby, I assumed, was a game for tough and hardy types, and was therefore ideal for 'real' or normal boys. Indeed, the teachers appeared to expect all us boys to play. Thus, I learnt that boys who did not play rugby were somehow not normal; that the boys who played soccer were, as we called them, poofs, but they were still better than those who didn't play any sports. And *those* boys deserved to be socially excluded from friendships and class activities.

Rugby's ability to operate as a prime dividing practice was, in part, closely orchestrated by my teachers. Throughout team selection processes we were subject to their gaze of authority and normalising judgement. Our sprinting abilities and other physical skills were routinely examined and recorded. Our bodily heights and weights were also measured and at times we were made to line up in order of shortest to tallest. These disciplinary techniques were used to classify us boys into three groups: 'A' and 'B' grade rugby players, and the abjects, the abnormals, or the others. These classifications helped objectify who we were according to the regimes of rugby and gender truths.

Further classification and surveillance occurred through the processes of my being selected for a provincial representative team. Those of us who made this team became discursively located in an even more privileged subject position, and throughout both primary and secondary school, as long as we continued to make the grade, we were treated venerably. We were, at times, driven in teachers' cars, invited to their houses, provided with ice-blocks when young and sometimes beer when older. We were given days off school and opportunities for trips nationally and internationally; teachers would look the other way if we were late to class and we were often given special help or dispensations with schoolwork. We were lauded in school assemblies, school newspapers, provincial newspapers and even on the radio. And as First XV high-school players, we even had a distinguishing school uniform, to help signify and reinforce our social status. Rugby therefore helped create subject positions, which gave us greater opportunities to speak and to be listened to. We became discursively located in influential positions to exercise power.

My youthful experiences of rugby are not unique. Recently many researchers have begun to examine the significance of school sport in the construction, negotiation and performance of dominant masculinities.[68] Skelton, for example, states that football, as central to the gender regime of the UK school she examined, 'defined relationships between males and females in the classroom and (even) took a central place in the classroom management strategies of the male teachers'.[69] Edley and Wetherell report, from the school they examined, that the most influential group in the sixth form was made up largely of the school's rugby players. They observed that a key aspect of their domination was physical:

> During breaktime, for instance, they would literally take over the common room with their boisterous games, forcing everyone else out on to the peripheries.

> Moreover, these games, like rugby, served to underline the players' ability to give and take physical punishment; a core aspect of the traditional definition of masculinity and a constant reminder of the threat posed to anyone wishing to challenge their dominant position.[70]

The overriding conclusion from these ethnographic studies is that schools are implicated in the construction of a gender regime that acts to advantage sporting boys.

THE DISCIPLINARY EFFECT OF RUGBY ON MY SENSE OF SELF

As a young man I could not escape the disciplinary powers associated with the dominating discursive practices of rugby and manliness. Although I was not directly coerced by some powerful group to act in a particular manner, I was soon tied to a subjectivity that was heavily shaped by rugby. Foucault states the body is 'directly involved in a political field; power relations have an immediate hold upon it; they invest it, mark it, train it, torture it, force it to carry out tasks, to perform ceremonies, to emit signs'.[71]

Indeed, the disciplinary power of rugby placed meticulous control on my bodily actions. I was careful who my friends were and what we talked about, and even how I sat or walked: my hands had to be in my pockets, my sleeves rolled up and my shirt hanging out. Occasionally I would feel compelled to spit. In fact, I became proficient at spitting; I would spit for accuracy, distance and style. I was also careful to hide certain emotions. I learnt at a young age not to cry in front of my peers, not to hug or sit too close to my male friends, and to distance myself from anything perceived as feminine, including my mum. Thus although as an eleven-year-old I still enjoyed sitting on my mum's knee at home or having her tuck me up in bed, I was careful not to be seen showing her affection in public. Likewise, I was particularly careful to hide my asthma. Asthma was a sign of weakness, so my inhaler was always carefully concealed at the bottom of my rugby gear bag. Nor did I let the boys know that I liked drama and cooking, or enjoyed playing the piano, and had once knitted a scarf.

Above all, it was important to be seen as tough and emotionally detached: walking to school on a cold morning in bare feet, although uncomfortable, was worth it. Similarly, one could never flinch in catching a high ball on the rugby field or avoid taking the tackle or being tackled; throwing a pass in desperation – a hospital pass, as we called it – was a sin.

Butler suggests that gender, as a performative technique of self, can be regarded as the 'repeated stylisation of the body, a set of repeated acts within a highly rigid regulatory frame that congeal over time to produce the appearance of substance, of a natural sort of being'.[72] Thus, the *performance* of these techniques of self took considerable practice to master, but eventually they felt natural.

Growing up and growing scared

By about the age of thirteen the dividing practices associated with rugby were starting to cause inner divisions. Specifically, I was becoming worried about getting physically hurt playing rugby, yet rugby men were meant to be tough and ignore pain. My coach would preach pre-game rhetoric such as 'the bigger they are, the harder they fall', or more usually 'hit them low around the legs and they'll come down'. However, I was concerned that my opponents were being indoctrinated by the same speeches.

To publicly criticise rugby was akin to criticising who we were, so a taboo of silence hung over this topic. Therefore I did not talk of my dislike for 'taking the tackle', or how I worried about being hurt, or that I hated being at the bottom of a ruck. And I didn't tell my teammates that before each game the threat of injury made me anxious, particularly if the opposition looked big and strong, as did my concern about letting the team down by missing a tackle or dropping a catch. Nor did I tell anyone that I disliked practising in the rain and mud, the laborious fitness drills of repeated sprints, sit-ups and press-ups where the last person was often singled out and made to do the drill again. In fact, the threat of being singled out was motivation enough to never be last. Upon recent reflection, I've become aware that my self-disciplinary rugby practices were motivated primarily by my desire to be accepted as 'normal'. However, the discourses that constituted normality within rugby were so specific, that although I was a normal rugby boy I was noticeably different from many other boys: at the time I judged this difference as 'superior'.

Strangely enough, although as a young teenager I worried in silence about being hurt in rugby, I had no qualms about inflicting pain on others. For example, I knew when running with the ball that it was entirely appropriate to pump my knees high and drop my shoulder into the opposition boy's chest or fend him forcefully in the face. And if I got to the try line and saw a boy lying on the ground, possibly hurt, I would actually feel good. I rationalised his pain as his fault; he was weak and unskilled, and this reaffirmed my strength and status. The discourses that constituted my violent actions in rugby also helped constitute my celebration of my opponent's pain.

Negotiation of meaning about pain and injury in rugby was never straightforward. Star reports that this negotiation process is complex, as two opposing discourses, each with ancestral history, permeate the game: 'fair' play or gentlemanly conduct versus 'fear' play or violence.[73] For example, I had to learn that a hard tackle around the chest that slammed the opposition to the ground, and caused pain, was good 'rugger'. However, a head high or stiff-arm tackle that slammed the opposition to the ground, and caused pain, was cowardly or dirty play. I also had to learn that motivations to 'kill or damage' the opposition during the game were entirely appropriate, but after the game the opposition became our new friends who we shook hands with and invited to share food and drink.

However, rugby was not all about risk-taking, violence and pain. The culture of the same did allow for the development of close and real male friendships. Rowe, for example, states that sport actually provides a legitimate space in which males can express feelings to each other, but homophobic attitudes act to rigidly limit the extent of such expression.[74] Yes indeed, my adolescence was a time when after scoring a try, even a pat on the back by a team-mate raised an eyebrow – there were no high fives and definitely no hugs. I even had to work hard at not smiling when running back to position after scoring a try. Displaying joyous emotion, unless drunk and celebrating a victory, was not something a rugby 'man' did.

As rugby culture was replete with multiple and competing discourses, it was at times difficult to negotiate consistent meaning from my teenage experiences with the game. However, I not only had to negotiate what was acceptable in rugby culture, I also had to make sense about whether what was appropriate in a rugby context was also appropriate in other social settings. It is perhaps not surprising that occasionally the divisions of what was acceptable on and off the rugby field blurred, particularly in all-male contexts. For example, the skills of physical intimidation glorified in rugby would at times be employed in physical education changing rooms or crowded school corridors, where smaller boys would be pushed to one side or out of the way.

Bullying and the threats of violence helped shape my early years at high school. I soon learnt where I could walk at lunchtime, whom I could talk to and whom to avoid; when it was appropriate to be intimidating and tough, and when this was a bad strategy. However, the discourses of rugby and manliness did not turn us all into violent and unitary men. Rob Hogan, for example, our biggest and undoubtedly toughest player in our high school First XV, would play as if demented or possessed, but was possibly the gentlest off the field. He was a silent type who enjoyed art, and I would often see him walking his little sister to kindergarten and kissing her goodbye; but with a rugby ball under his arm he was a sadistic, pain-inflicting machine.

Living the contradictions

The competing discourses that surrounded rugby and the more general discourses associated with being a respectful or ethical individual impacted on my subjectivity and I lived, unbeknown to myself, a life of contradictions. Possibly the largest contradiction I was living occurred in the last two years of high school, when I started to think of myself as gentle and sensitive to others. I took pride in the fact that I had never been in a 'real' physical fight; and, although a decade too late, I was influenced by the anti-war and protest music of Bob Dylan and John Lennon. I was beginning to view myself as some sort of junior peace-loving hippy. This self-image did not gel well with pre-game pep talks by our captain who often said: 'Remember, we're a team and we all support each other. If there's a fight, we're all in. We don't let a team mate down.' Yet, I was only vaguely aware of these contradictions. I should have been aware of the contradictions the day the 1981 Springboks played Nelson Bays. I walked down the main street protesting against apartheid and violence, and then slipped away from the protest action into Trafalgar Park to watch the game. I particularly wanted to see my high school coach play. He had told me it would be the biggest thrill of his life playing the South Africans.

Nevertheless, I was acutely aware of the tensions caused by my fear of injury with the expectations that 'real' rugby men are tough and ignore pain. But I did not want to simply quit rugby as my sense of self was still closely tied to the game. Indeed, as a member of the First XV I was actively using rugby as a 'technique of self' for my own advantages. However, this was a time when resistance to the dominance of rugby in New Zealand was at its pinnacle. The disastrous 1981 South African Springbok tour had sparked massive anti-racist and anti-rugby protests. These protests 'unleashed a depth of public feeling and civil unrest in New Zealand unmatched since the Depression'.[75] For a time, these protests promoted a reverse discourse which acted to position rugby players as politically ignorant, sexist and violent.

This competing discourse helped legitimate my concerns with the pain of rugby but also added to my inner tensions. Before rugby games I often asked myself: 'Why am I playing this ridiculous game?' and after games, particularly if my body was bruised and sore, I would ask similar questions. By the time I got to university, as an eighteen-year-old, these alternative discursive resources gave me the strength to quit playing rugby; but it was more difficult to completely reject the game.

Epilogue

Even today, although I'm now highly critical of the place of rugby in New Zealand society, the dominating discourses of rugby and manliness still impact on me and I find it difficult to fully escape their disciplinary power and live a life free of contradiction, tension and fragmentation.

For example, toward the end of a recent lecture in which I vigorously critiqued the place of rugby in Aotearoa, I noticed several of the students, mainly males, looking disgruntled. I subsequently started to feel uneasy, almost unpatriotic, as if I were somehow letting 'my side' down. The pressure finally got to me and in my closing statements, I relented: 'Hey, rugby's not all bad. I use to play the game and quite enjoyed aspects of it.' And then, using nationalism (a major dividing practice), I made a weak attempt at humour: 'And of course I still support two teams, the All Blacks and any team playing the Wallabies'.

After class I thought through what had happened. By being critical of rugby I had felt personally threatened. In response I turned, once again, to the dominance of rugby to help legitimise my stance and to defend myself, or more specifically, to defend my manliness. By stating I had once played rugby and still enjoyed watching the New Zealand *men's* team, I had used rugby to try and show I was a normal man. The disciplinary effect of rugby and its dividing and normalising practices were still influential.

Although my rugby story does not end with a tidy concluding statement about my sense of self, through this Foucauldian examination I have realised the powerful effect of dominating discourses. This recognition inspires me to further examine and challenge the dominating discourses that link rugby union and other combat-style sports with particular masculinities.

I thank Pirkko Markula, Wendy Drewery and Louisa Allen for helpful comments on an earlier draft of this paper.

four

Managing the Margins: Gay-Disabled Masculinity

TERRY O'NEILL

In contrast to the ways in which they are commonly understood or represented, gender, sexuality and impairment are not now, nor ever have been, either neutral or necessarily 'scientific' concepts. Rather, they are perhaps more usefully approached as quite particular and malleable forms of subjective and social experience much influenced by their discursive articulation in specific historical eras. They are not, then, static or objective descriptors but arise as periodic convergences of meaning and significance. In this discussion the subjective and social categories of 'masculine', 'disabled' and 'homosexual' are approached according to the view that they are constituted and reconstituted as particular – and highly particularising – epochal convergences of 'truth' and 'knowledge'.

While all men are susceptible to the impermanence of these meanings across time, gay-disabled men are often particularly sensitised to the conjuncture of definitions with social and subjective context. For these men, contemporaneously hegemonic notions of the 'truth' and 'reality' of masculinity emerge as complex subjective matters involving aspiration and disappointment, conditional success and sometimes personally devastating failure. The dominant subjective and social meanings against which these struggles of the marginalised and sometimes divided self occur, are those associated with heterosexual masculinity and unimpaired male physicality. This is the discursive and ideological terrain within which the gay-disabled male is first brought into being, and subsequently maintained, as the personification of negative difference; as the embodiment of distinctive forms of 'abnormality' and 'pathology' relative to the idealised and explicitly normalised heterosexual and able-bodied male subject.

The appreciation by the gay-disabled that they are in some important respects *different* also entails – over the course of individual life histories – the gradual accumulation of an array of supplementary 'knowledges'. Primary among these is the comprehension that considerably more discursive and social power is ascribed to those configurations of meanings which are unambiguously dedicated to the validation of the 'norm'. In other words, both male impairment and homosexuality are implicated in a web of power relations within which they are generally deemed to be negative male characteristics. Under these conditions the social, ideological, political, and embodied differences entailed by male gay-disability may ensure that its *experience* becomes coincidental with quite specific subjective appreciations of the ways in which power operates in contemporary Western societies.

The claim that modern power is both complex and diffuse is today a relatively typical analytical premise. The discussion which follows is perhaps less concerned with re-emphasising this now generally accepted view than with describing a specific social and subjective context in which 'power' can and does emerge as a highly unpredictable concept and an often 'unreadable' dimension of individual and/or collective experience. For gay-disabled men, an experiential as well as an analytic tension emerges between the social power ascribed to males generally and the implications for those individuals who fail to meet the prescriptive ideological expectations circulated by hegemonic masculinity and its various discourses. More than most men, gay-disabled men face the challenge of subjectively validating – and making some sense of – an array of sometimes contradictory historical and contemporary discourses and discursive practices around what, exactly, it means to be a man in the twenty-first century. In this respect, gay-disabled men are often distinguishable from hegemonic forms of masculinity simply by the relative complexity of their understandings of the sometimes contradictory ways in which masculine power affects individual and collective experience. In short, and not least because they often articulate knowledge of the ways in which power can be simultaneously enabling and constraining, the gay-disabled man emerges as an uncommonly rich source for the investigation of the myriad dimensions of forms of modern power.

It is tempting to at least partially attribute the dearth of research into gay-disabled masculinity to the inherent complexity of this form of male difference. Alternatively, and pertinently to any discussion of power and its operation(s), it could also be claimed that the analytic silences which have for so long been a feature of gay-disabled male experience are themselves one outcome of the historical trajectory of hegemonic discourses relating to masculinity and to intra-masculine relations. This is to observe that, for more years than has been warranted, a unitary representation of masculinity has reigned with almost unquestioned supremacy within the social and other sciences. The academic and social dominance of these meanings has not been without implication for gay-disabled men and, it might be suggested, may even have contributed to aspects of their continued subordination. Indeed, many gay-disabled men have struggled with the lack of resemblance, indeed the lack of relevance, that theoretical pronouncements about masculinity have to their own experience.

For these men, the continued signification of unitary and undifferentiated theories of male gender may provide a powerful basis for individual subjective dissonance. Nevertheless, and somewhat belatedly, one of the more significant tendencies in contemporary studies of masculinity has been the evident intellectual and ideological 'slippage' of the once indisputably hegemonic unitary interpretation of masculinity. Within this new climate of enquiry it is becoming increasingly acceptable to question the integrity, and the motives, of longstanding attempts to assign all men collective attributes to the level of social structure. This is to at last acknowledge that gay-disabled men – either individually or in diverse forms of collectivity – are now, just as they always have been, involved in the authentication of subjectively coherent masculinities which have always existed as forms of differentiated and marginalised male experience. In other words, it is to resignify the lived individual experience of masculinity and to emphatically acknowledge that masculinities are first lived and then theorised.

Very clearly then, and not least because gender theory has most usually failed both gay-disabled subjectivities and experience in the past, this is to signify experience over theory and to centralise the emphases and contradictions articulated by gay-disabled men themselves. This discussion draws, then, upon data collected during interviews with fifteen gay-disabled men who, themselves, represent a diverse cohort stratified by age, socio-economic status, and the individualising implications of their own impairment. Embodying a wide variety of both congenital and acquired conditions ranging from psychiatric through to mobility or both, or sensory impairment, the respondents were differentiated by the subjective and social significances attached to their own disability, but all approached the research on the basis of their self-identification as both homosexual and physically impaired male subjects. The interviews in which these men participated were necessarily semi-structured events designed to accommodate their individual capacities and subjective emphases while, simultaneously, allowing for the collection of data relating to previously identified themes and areas of collective investigative interest. Although thematic constancies in the respondents' accounts naturally provided a significant organisational basis for the analysis, this did not occur at the expense of ignoring or subordinating instances of individual inconsistency, contradiction, or exceptional 'unruliness'. Rather, the experiential differences which emerged in the interviews were often the source of important insights into gay-disabled masculinities.

The gay-disabled man and subjective dissonance

Like all subjects, gay-disabled men are much concerned with the notion and accomplishment of subjective reconciliation and coherent identity. They are, then, implicated in the pervasive and longstanding philosophical concern for subjectivity as an aspect of the fabrication of the citizen-subject and his relation to the social order.[1] For multiply-differentiated males, however, this is a complex aspiration made consistently more difficult by the susceptibility of 'identity' to forms of reductionism and over-simplification.[2] So while there is a general social tendency to at least conditionally authenticate the identities of 'disabled' and 'gay', this occurs against a conceptual and ideological intransigence which continues to imply that their subjective and/or identificatory *convergence* is implausible.

Notwithstanding that they are disadvantaged by unitary understandings of identity, gay-disabled men must nonetheless attempt to position themselves relative to the manifest significances attached – in all times and in all places – to the subjective and social project entailed in the formulation of both individual and collective identity. A formative element of the wider aspiration towards effective identification is the extensive discursive repertoire concerned with the ways of being and acting – the forms of psychic and physical reality or 'truth' – which are deemed to underpin both male subjectivity and subject-position. These discourses range from the still hegemonic interpretation of authentic masculinity as being both heterosexual and unimpaired to the more recent forms of discursive 'counter-power' claimed by the politics of difference and marginalised identity. Irrespective of their individual emphases, these discourses share common features which ensure that the male body is maintained as both a topic and an object of power. Consequently, gay-disabled men are consistently enjoined to signify their bodies, and especially the functional and performative aspects of their bodies, as matters of central subjective, social and political interest.

These constituted dispositions are of complex and often longstanding origin. For gay-disabled men, as for other men, the institutionalised family emerges as an enduring referential complex concerned with the dissemination of understandings around both hetero-normative masculinity and the legitimate (implicitly able-bodied) expression of male gender. In its constituted role as a powerful discursive and subjective influence, the family draws upon and – in diverse forms of reciprocity – also conditions supplementary discourses around 'normal' (customarily, Christian) ethics and morality as well as normative modes of education and styles of inter-personal relationships. For multiply-differentiated men, however, the influence of family life is seldom limited to the constitution of individual appreciations around the centrality of 'authentic' masculinity to coherent male subjectivity. Rather, it extends to the conditioned and early appreciation that the two differences which they embody are susceptible to quite contrasting interpretations and responses. Thus, while the hetero-normativity of families and other institutions emerges a consistently negative and regulating feature of their homosexual experience, gay-disabled men can often signify the family as a site of relative *tolerance* around their impairment. This discursive capacity to discern between male differences – to attribute relative values to male difference – can, for gay-disabled men, emerge as an enduring element of their experiences within the supplementary contexts of employment, medicine, and both sexual and non-sexual relationships.

In these and other ways, gay-disabled men learn to recognise themselves as subjects who may simultaneously correspond with *and* contravene both the embodiment and the accomplishment of authentic and/or exemplary masculinity. The very ambiguity of this position presents a subjective locale which may be construed by self and others in a variety of ways and according to a variety of understandings around the subjective and social implications of difference itself. However, gay-disabled men are most usually understood to be at least partially – and sometimes completely – aberrant, counterfeit, nonsensical or dissonant gender entities. This outcome reflects the continued dominance of the hegemonic construct as well as its intractability towards male difference.

Viewed against the discursive complex relating to the variety of ways in which it might be deemed possible to be male, gay-disabled men are at once subjectively and socially constituted as simultaneously plausible (comprehensible) *and* contradictory (incomprehensible) by the conditions of their multiple relations to power and its operation. Theirs is, then, a subject-position produced in the continual interaction between discourses and subjectivity; a relationship between the subject and discourse which may be experienced as contradictory, oppositional,[3] or inherently unstable.[4] Centrally, the gay-disabled man is constituted at the point of intersection of a multiplicity of subject-positions whose interrelations may themselves be the result of hegemonic practices.[5]

Because gay-disabled men are customarily and increasingly maintained in negative relation to power and its operation(s), they are commonly implicated in equivalently subordinated forms of representation and conditioned subjective and social experience. Subjectivities do not compete equally but are themselves implicated in struggles to have particular ways of being a man privileged or taken for the norm so that subjectivities are a site of struggle and change rather than fixed, homogeneous and enduring.[6] Under these conditions, male gay-disability subjectivity is experienced physically, through practices which are simultaneously physical *and* discursive.[7] In other words, it is possible – and even likely – that gay-disabled men will assign markedly contrasting implications or potentials to the differences they embody. Indeed, one of the earliest insights provided by the men who participated in this study was their evident disposition to interpret or experience (or both) the convergence of their homosexuality and disability as a sometimes debilitating form of subjective dissonance. This is not to suggest that the respondents avoided any subjective alignment with their differences *per se*. Rather, it is to note that they almost uniformly privileged the psychic integration of just one difference over the simultaneous or equivalent integration of *both* differences. A complex subjective undertaking, this process of subjective resolution to one comparatively validated difference was often acknowledged by the men in the study to be a tenuous enterprise and, at times, a conditional achievement. Indeed, and as if to emphasise the potential of multiple-differentiation to continue to contribute to individual subjective dissonance, even the validated difference remained susceptible to the ever-present subjective and social implications of the subordinated difference.

It is, then, the complex subjective inscription of gay-disabled men which forms the basis of their disposition towards the maintenance of equivalently diffuse connections with forms of modern power. However, these connections are not without irony or subjective contradiction. On the one hand, and notwithstanding their capacity to periodically engage with key aspects of the hegemonic construct, the respondents' accounts were replete with instances in which the subjective and social distance between meta-theoretical claims and the details of their lived experience could arise as powerful points of contention and indignation. Many reacted with derision to any suggestion that their masculinity automatically provided them with universal economic, social and sexual benefits. Others provided disturbing accounts of their explicit regulation – most commonly directed at their homosexuality – by apparently heterosexual males. However, while the men in this study could readily identify hegemonic (unimpaired and heterosexual) males as their subordinating other, they nonetheless generally considered hegemonic masculinity to be more or less synonymous with the operations and interests of modern social power. Thus, for a number of the respondents, the maintenance of their productive connections with hegemonic male power emerged as a matter of on-going interest, and was often reflected in a concern with the relative 'visibility' or 'invisibility' of their differences. To this extent, without exception and often heavily dependent upon specific contexts, all the respondents simultaneously maintained and enacted complex forms of both hegemonic *and* marginalised masculinity.

Male difference and counter-power

Gay-disabled men necessarily share with all other subjects a constituted desire to comprehend the terms of their relations to modern forms of power. In this respect, gay-disabled men can be particularly motivated by the contemporary interest in forms of existence and understanding which are more purposefully relative to multiply-differentiated and multiply-located subjects. Indeed, given the extent of their constituted subjective and social dissonance, the aspiration for coherent subjectivity might be assumed to hold new potentials for those gay-disabled men who recognise that the forms and implications of the differential operation of power have given rise to multiple masculinities.[8]

Nevertheless, and as I have already noted, gay-disabled men customarily maintain forms of complicity with the hegemonic construct which could profoundly complicate their own attempts to construe themselves as uniformly or consistently oppressed by heterosexual and/or able-bodied males. While their physical or emotional vulnerability to the activities and responses of hegemonic males may provide them with the basis of a critique of hetero-normative masculinity, other aspects of their activities and attitudes imply more complex forms of subjective relationship with the dominant construct. For instance, and in marked contrast to their low opinion of apparently 'feminised' gay men, the respondents in this study almost uniformly signified the demeanours and attributes associated with hegemonic masculinity. Further, these dispositions could extend from their occasional complicity in the subordination of other marginalised men to the purposeful emulation of hegemonic male characteristics in both 'heterosexual' *and* 'homosexual' contexts. Thus, and virtually irrespective of social context, authentic male gender performance is maintained as consistent preoccupation. Indeed, tensions which exist between the respondents' critique of hegemonic masculinity and their simultaneous propensity to emulate it emerge as potentially confounding features of their accounts.

It is these aspects of gay-disabled male experience which provide a further indication that the previously hegemonic meta-narrative of undifferentiated masculinity provides a very limited analytic context within which the convergence of male impairment and homosexuality might be explored. In paradoxical emulation of the extent to which heterosexual and able-bodied men are encouraged to imagine themselves to be uniformly empowered, to construe gay-disabled men as similarly disempowered is to fundamentally misinterpret this subject-position. Rather, it may be that for both 'hegemonic' and 'marginalised' men the reality of their respective relations to power and its operation(s) might be more usefully thought of as rather more similar than different. In short, while gay-disabled men are often construed by themselves and others as uniformly and differentially (negatively) empowered, as unambiguously marginalised, it remains that a dichotomous characterisation of their relations with hegemonic male power is seldom, if ever, reliable.

The assertion that gay-disabled men are maintained in a complex relationship to power and its operation(s) is not a particularly meaningful insight. Rather, and because gay-disabled men can at different times articulate alternately simple *and* complex understandings of power, what emerges as a matter of associated interest are those specific discursive, subjective, political and social contexts which posit the view that power is neither a complex nor multidimensional concept. In other words, gay-disabled men *are* uniformly subordinated on the basis of their homosexuality or impairment. More particularly, a primary analytic interest occurs around those discourses and/or political or identity convergences which apparently articulate a correspondence between meaningful and resistant forms of counter-power and explicitly dichotomous interpretations of power.

The politics of male difference

As I have already noted, gay-disabled men are clearly disposed to validate one of their differences over the other. An important part of their explanations around this subjective and identificatory strategy rests upon their evident capacity to legitimate some aspects of the primary but often disparate discourses (both hegemonic and marginalised) which are available to them while explicitly rejecting others. Indeed, this must necessarily be recognised as a significant aspect of the complex subjective project which arises when multiply-differentiated males undertake the identification of the discourse(s) and subject-position(s) which are most aligned with their interests. Thus, and in all circumstances, gay-disabled men must attempt to reconcile the 'fusion of cultural meaning with personal emotional meaning that is tied to the psycho-biographical history of any individual'.[9] While the propensity of gay-disabled men to subscribe to, and articulate, elements from a range of discourses is a likely outcome of their multi-situationality, neither is this without implication for the ways in which they formulate subjective and social identity. In other words, since they must strategise in the continued absence of any incorporative counter-discourse which conjoins both male disability *and* homosexuality, this also means that their constitution of subjectively meaningful marginalised identities and forms of counter-power is effectively restricted to either the discourses of disability or male homosexuality. This limitation of identificatory choice stands in contrast to the ways in which gay-disabled men understand power to be both differential and contextual so that important subjective reservations can impede the unconditional alignment by individuals with the forms of counter-power claimed by either disability or gay identity. Indeed, unconditional alignment with just *one* marginalised identity can become a potentially problematic and/or contradictory strategy.

In common with all other politics, the politics of male difference are a terrain of individual and collective scrutiny, contention, discursive competition and, occasionally, interventionist therapeutics. In order to reflect this complexity, this analysis draws upon a conceptualisation of power which emphasises its disparate and sometimes contradictory interests. Here, power is characterised – in *all* of its formations – as purposefully and simultaneously enabling and constraining so that no dimension of gay-disabled male experience is held to be removed from its pervading influences and diverse interests. While this form of analysis rejects any understanding of the subject-position of the gay-disabled man as a uniform metaphor for marginalisation, it does not discount or devalue instances of marginalisation. Rather, it serves to emphasise the point that even apparently emancipatory configurations of marginalised male identity and politics are not immune from either the effects or the sometimes obscure objectives of hegemonic male power.

This observation is nowhere more evident than in the frequency with which the respondents in this study could point to instances of their own oppression within the contexts of the politics of difference. Thus, on the one hand, gay-disabled men are commonly exposed to explicit or implicit ableism in gay settings while, on the other hand, they can also experience unexpected and equally destructive homophobia in disability contexts. Indeed, by way of example, just one of the respondents in this study believed that the disability community unconditionally accepted his homosexuality. The much more common experience was that the disclosure of homosexuality within disability settings entailed similar – or even *more* considered – levels of premeditation and evaluation than relatively hegemonic contexts.

These events, and the understandings which they generated, can emphasise for gay-disabled men the evident and constituted implausibility of one difference when it is expressed in the context of the other difference. In turn, this might suggest that gay-disabled 'agency', as well as the marginalised identities with which it might be associated, emerges as a conditioned and conditional concept suffused with the dual power to both enable and constrain individuals. More controversially, it might construe identity politics as having the unavoidable potential to act upon the acting and multiply-differentiated marginalised subject in explicitly negative ways. Even more disconcertingly, this is to suggest that marginalised political contexts emulate hegemonic contexts to the extent that they maintain a discernible interest not only in subjective coercion but also in effective forms of self-surveillance and self-correction to perversely marginalised 'norms'.[10] Clearly, such an understanding of the pervasiveness of power entails the corresponding view that even marginality is available for reconfiguration into new forms of orthodoxy. Further, and in contrast to its superficial emancipatory connotations, this is to comprehend politics of difference as formations which engage with individuals and groups as both technologies of domination *and* technologies of the self to facilitate governance of the self under less authoritative forms of modern power[11] 'beyond the state';[12] a sustaining and individualising art of government underpinned by forms of modern 'self-identity'.[13]

Although there is evidence of a proliferation of new discourses relating to those subjects now coded as 'marginalised' or 'excluded',[14] both subjective and political realities continue to be largely defined for marginalised men by hegemonic formations so that new discursive formations can be closely associated with new strategies of governance. In common with all subjects, gay-disabled men are enjoined into self-governance by means of a set of technologies so that the conduct of government becomes linked to the government of conduct.[15] This raises the somewhat distasteful possibility that marginalised formations are sites of simultaneous emancipation *and* regulation for gay-disabled men. In other words, they are implicated in the intensification of interventions linked to the multiplication of interlocking discourses all of which are tightly articulated around a cluster of power relations.[16]

The gay-disabled man has arisen as the embodiment of new knowledges, new modes of power and as the subject and object of new modes of control over the bodies, consciousness and identity of human beings.[17] According to this view, hegemonic masculinity must be interpreted as just one aspect of the complex operation of power in which the constitution and maintenance of gay-disabled individuals as marginalised and docile citizens remain a central objective. Because power is established, consolidated and implemented in the functioning of discourse and thus brings into being complex relations between groups, forms of dissonance and incoherence are evident in all forms of subjective and/or political affiliation. Thus, while the new identities of the current era can offer self-actualisation they can also lead to fragmentation, insecurity and powerlessness,[18] so that they might be both emblematic of the diffusion of norms as well as the constitution of new forms of control.[19]

It is possible, then, that the politics of difference can operate as obscure, but nonetheless explicit, sites of complex and diffuse regulation of the multiply-differentiated marginalised male subject. Indeed, in this respect, the emancipatory potentials of the conventional identity politics, which underpin both homosexuality and disability, are held by many gay-disabled men to be constitutively limited in the extent to which they could accommodate multiple male differentiation. Rather, both the gay and disability communities play a complex and sometimes paradoxical role in the formulation of coherent identity for gay-disabled males.

Organising gay-disabled male identity

While two distinct primary marginalised identities are available to gay-disabled men in the current era, the men who participated in this study almost uniformly privileged their homosexual identity over their identity as impaired individuals. Very clearly, and notwithstanding evidence of their subjective dissonance, the personal identificatory strategy represented by the hierarchisation of their marginalised identities was generally understood by the respondents to be a valid and productive strategy.

In some important ways, the ordering of marginalised identities by male gay-disabled adults presents a marked contrast to attempts – by self or others – to manage personal identity in their juvenile or even pre-adolescent life-stages.

As if to emphasise the point that personal identity arises as an 'issue' in both 'apolitical' as well as explicitly 'political' contexts, many respondents drew upon often longstanding memories of their socialisation within the family and other institutions. Indeed, their experience of family and family life was often used as the basis for a related thematic emphasis upon the ways in which *others* purposefully discriminate between the identities of disabled and homosexual. Thus, gay-disabled men's experience of the potentially problematic convergence of homosexuality with impairment can emerge as a set of often deeply insightful appreciations. First constructed within the contexts of family, school, work and friendships, any or all of these understandings may have preceded 'political' consciousness in any commonly accepted sense.

Particularly with respect to their homosexuality, the understanding that the interpersonal and social responses to male impairment and homosexuality can be similar but also markedly different can have important subjective implications for gay-disabled males. Early life and experience provided respondents in this study with the complex and perhaps subjectively foundational knowledge that different types and styles of male bodies can be implicated in relations of power in distinctly contrasting ways. Or, that while both identities are objects of widespread subordination relative to power and its operation(s), it is the identity of the male homosexual which commonly provokes a relatively more thoroughgoing sense of familial and social consternation. In later life, and as very many gay-disabled men can attest, the negative potentiality of 'homosexual male' can ensure that the subjective and lived experience of homosexuality is often structured by the interpersonal and institutional violences exerted against it. Under these conditions, and in virtually all life-stages, the disclosure of homosexuality can arise as a matter of great personal significance and, potentially, as a crucial influence over identificatory strategies and the accomplishment of subjective coherence.

Although the men in this study described generally less intransigent family attitudes towards their disability compared to their homosexuality, both forms of difference could be interpreted as contradictory to the family's understanding that authentic masculinity is necessarily heterosexual and able-bodied. Customarily, male impairment is comprehended and evaluated in relation to the implied strength and perfection of the image of the male body inferred by the dominating discursive influence of the hegemonic construct of masculinity. As the congenitally impaired respondents in this study could attest, the family is an important but often restricted source of information about the impaired male body. The significances attached to 'normal' male functionality can be evident in the forms of physical discernment employed by the family and may extend to the articulation by families of a range of 'normalising' discourses and strategies around appropriate medical interventions and styles of education. Under these circumstances, the manifestation of male impairment can be a source of consternation and effrontery. Even more, it can form the basis of personal interpretations around the coincidences that might exist between male impairment and gender-transgression.

Male impairment may so confound the implicit expectations of the family as to result in the effective termination of ties of intimacy and/or 'normal' inter-personal engagement. However, the respondents in this study did not construe the family as uniformly unhelpful in the matter of their disability. Much more commonly, the family was understood as a discursive and experiential setting within which there was an evident concern with 'coming to terms' with their impairment. Significantly, this could stand in marked contrast to the family's frequent unwillingness to acknowledge or explore issues around homosexuality.

While gay-disabled men consistently emphasise the centrality of early experience to their understanding of both their homosexuality and impairment, the respondents also indicated that their subjective and social emphases could change markedly following their transition as adults into wider socio-economic relations. The impaired male body's positioning in more or less consistently negative relation to power and its operation(s) is evidence of the general tendency to purposefully construe impaired male bodies as power-deficit entities. Thus, and again emulating the subjectively conditioning effects of the social response to their homosexuality, the disclosure of impairment emerges as a distinctly significant matter for many gay-disabled males – particularly, perhaps, for those men with 'invisible' disabilities. Moreover, the assumption of a disability identity is often held to be further complicated both by the type of impairment and the evident subjective hierarchisation of a range of different impairments.

Notwithstanding that those men with 'visible' impairment have little choice that they are made available for identification by others as disabled, the disclosure by individuals of their homosexuality and/or disability is a salient and necessarily repetitive subjective and social exercise. Further, disclosure can be understood in complex ways. As, for instance, both emblematic of negative positionality relative to power and its operation as well as a manifestation of counter-power. However, and notwithstanding that in contemporary contexts disclosure (or 'coming out') is often viewed as a necessary prerequisite to the constitution of coherent subjectivity and identity, disclosure for gay-disabled men can be highly problematic. It can, for instance, mean that their self-identification to others can result in either the disjuncture of existing relationships – both social and economic – or even verbal or physical assault.

These, then, are the circumstances within which gay-disabled men simultaneously experience identification as both a disciplinary project as well as a form of potential counter-power or resistance. Given that their identification as either homosexual or as disabled can emerge as an ongoing and risk-laden subjective and social enterprise, the more or less uniform validation of homosexual identity over disabled identity by gay-disabled men raises several questions. Not the least of these is that very often gay identity is a less than accommodating context for the subjective and social articulation of any form of male impairment. Indeed, and notwithstanding that some respondents – and particularly those with 'invisible' impairments – could go to considerable lengths to accomplish its authentic imitation, the 'hyper-masculine' emphasis often associated with gay culture, community and politics was consistently derided by the men in this study. They could, for instance, relate numerous instances of their own experience to support the view that this bodily ideal remained unattainable for many disabled men and was, more often than not, itself a source of continued subjective dissonance.

These experiences in gay contexts stand in marked contrast to the numerous ways in which the respondents in this study consistently centralised the accomplishment of intimacy as a matter of profound and ongoing concern. Notwithstanding that they were susceptible to subordination in both disability and gay settings, they were much inclined to construe these contexts in markedly different ways. So while homosexual identity was much more commonly held to have the potential to facilitate the accomplishment of intimacy, disability identity was not. Thus, sexual encounters arising from gay clubs and sex-on-site venues emerge as matters of primary subjective and identificatory interest because they are also contexts in which the inherent tensions between the identities of gay men and disabled men may be most explicitly evident. Often, the negative experience of the convergence of these identities can politicise gay-disabled men in quite particular ways. They are, for instance, very much more inclined to subscribe to an individualised gay identity rather than to engage with gay politics in its collectivised or ostensibly 'political' formations.

Nevertheless, and despite their frequent acknowledgement that the idealised male body was a regulatory dimension of their experience, the erotic appeal of unimpaired male physicality was seldom explicitly dismissed or even discounted by the informants in this study. Rather, it emerged in their accounts as a referential sign and as a way of being and acting against which they evaluated themselves and against which they felt that they were evaluated by others. To this extent, the discursive and experiential relationships which are maintained between exemplary masculinity and gay-disabled subjectivity might be more usefully understood as necessarily complex; as, perhaps, indicative of the ways in which power operates in formations which involve both forms of domination *and* as particularising disciplines of the self.

In some important ways the accounts upon which this discussion is based are cautionary. They indicate that, even within multiply-differentiated and marginalised male subjectivities, hegemonic and exemplary masculinity is nonetheless maintained as an organising – and individualising – aspiration. This suggests that, particularly for those men with 'visible' impairment, their preferred identity contributes little substantive opportunity for them to be construed as sexually desirable – or even sexual – subjects. In large part, this again reflects the negative positioning of male impaired bodies within networks of power and the extent to which such bodies are construed as effectively power-deficit and so susceptible to interpretation as both gender-less (or gender neutral) or sexuality-less. These tendencies, often arrayed around specific types of disability or degrees of individual impairment, stand in thoroughgoing contrast, and tension, to the ways in which unimpaired bodies are understood to be – essentially, unalterably, consistently *and* necessarily – 'naturally' gendered and sexualised. In this sense, and as the object *and* the terrain of an array of discourses and discursive practices among which its gender and its sexuality are explicated as conditional rather than essential attributes, the impaired male body is maintained as an inherently – subjectively and socially – deficient concept and form of experience.

The more or less uniform privileging of their gay over their disability identity is, I suggest, primarily motivated by the ideological and political correspondences which are perceived to exist between gay identification and the hegemonic reification of the unimpaired male body as both authentically desirable *and* as potentially powerful. Notwithstanding that gay-disabled men are markedly less likely to achieve the accomplishment of intimacy in disability settings, the gay contexts with which gay-disabled males must necessarily engage represent often unhelpful ideological and subjective convergences for the resolution of dissonance. Nevertheless, to the extent that they are clearly disposed towards the hierarchisation of the various identities available to them as multiply-differentiated subjects, gay-disabled men appear to continue to rely upon many of the same understandings evident in wider society of the relationships maintained between identity and power and its operation(s). Thus, and beginning with their complex, often conflictual, but subjectively affirming engagement with the hegemonic construct of masculinity, gay-disabled males often appear to draw upon and replicate those same hegemonic understandings of masculinity which contribute so strongly to their own regulation and subjective dissonance.

Conclusions

One of the defining features of the experience of the convergence of disability and homosexuality is that one form of difference is very often negatively regulated by the political-identificatory articulation of the other. Thus, few of the respondents in this study could report that they had achieved the successful subjective or social reconciliation of one difference within the political or community context of the other. Indeed, and arising from instances of their own experience, the politics of difference are often interpreted by gay-disabled men with suspicion and some trepidation as – variously – personally inauthentic or even 'unsafe'.

The achievement of unconflicted identity is, under these circumstances, a potentially problematic aspiration. Nevertheless, its resolution is discursively and politically construed as both possible and desirable – as something which might be 'worked on' and 'worked through' within the context of ostensibly resistant politics of difference. According to this interpretation, new formations of collectivised marginalised identity are held to denote points of conflict between a declining but still vigorous system of domination and subordination and newly emergent forms of opposition.[20] However, male gay-disabled experience suggests that the ostensibly emancipatory 'knowledges' and roles articulated by the politics of difference operate according to quite diffuse imperatives when faced with the multiple-differentiation of potential constituents. The propensity for these politics to functionally contribute to the subjective dissonance – which gay-disabled men understand is, itself, a rationale for their affiliation – seems clear. Instead, these men often experience these politics as being more emphatically concerned with the terms of the relationships between their organising difference and hegemonic power rather than with the amelioration or resolution of either inter-difference or inter-masculine relations. Under these conditions, then, it is possible that the politics of difference may be at least partially conducive to the continued hegemony of both normative physicality and sexuality.

So far as disability politics are concerned, the respondents in this study could apparently affirm some ideological/political aspects of disability identity, such as discrimination, while explicitly rejecting others. However, and notwithstanding that there is indeed a clear correlation between disability-based discrimination and power restriction, they were not generally inclined to accept these correspondences as evidence that their masculinity had been compromised by their impairment. Rather, they could commonly understand disability identity as a *contravention* of key aspects of their masculinity.

Given their almost uniform propensity to privilege their homosexual identity, it is somewhat paradoxical that some men in this study could suggest that disability identity was the more socially acceptable. Nevertheless, while most (although not all) were prepared to accept the relevance of the term 'disabled' as a personal descriptor (to acknowledge that they were impaired in some way), just two were prepared to name disability as an 'identity' in a collectivised sense. In contrast, but again exhibiting the general tendency to eschew the communal or politicised identities articulated by either formation, the balance of the sample preferenced their individual rather than collectivised identity as relatively 'non-political' and markedly conditional 'communal' gay males.

Commonly, the decision to interpret their homosexuality as an individualising rather than a collectivising strategy was associated with instances of their explicit impairment-based oppression or rejection in gay contexts. So, in common with their experience of disability contexts, gay-disabled males' engagement with gay community or politics could apparently be a dissembling and internally alienating strategy.

However, gay-disabled men strongly imply that their aspiration to accomplish forms and events of inter-personal intimacy is a conditioning aspect of their willingness to negotiate (or endure) negative responses to their impairment in gay social/sexual settings. In direct contrast to the potential for their accomplishment of intimacy, which they could associate with the exemplary masculinity reified by gay politics, they could also understand that the politics of disability is – necessarily – concerned with the *relegation* of aesthetic male physicality rather than its consistent and potentially erotic exemplification. Under these subjective and discursive conditions, heterosexual disability politics cannot very easily be construed by gay-disabled males as a viable or enduring context either for sexual practice, or for the precursive physical-erotic values which they signify as the objects of their aspirations around intimacy.

At both the personal and political levels the objective of stable and coherent multiply-situated male identity is evidently experienced as a sometimes traumatic and inherently problematic ambition. Notwithstanding their frequent attempts to achieve subjective and identificatory reconciliation, the gay-disabled men who participated in this study frequently described instances of their implicit or explicit oppression when one difference was articulated within the context of the other, and when *either* difference arose in relation to the hegemonic construct of masculinity. Given these subjective and discursive parameters, it would appear that gay-disabled males almost uniformly manage the aspiration to coherent, stable and unconflicted identity by means of a complex and potentially problematic strategy involving the subjective subordination of one marginalised identity to the other. The details of their accounts, however, imply that this strategy is seldom without subjective or social implications, so that identity issues are often the continued source of deep and consistent introspection over time. This suggests that despite their signification of gay identity, the details of male gay-disabled experience belie any attempt to construe this strategy as wholly effective or even functionally coherent. Rather, the convergence of disability with homosexuality is very commonly experienced as a source of manifest tensions, which themselves continue to negatively structure the subjective and social relations which exist between the subject's primary and subordinated identities.

This is, perhaps, evidence of the extent and embeddedness of the subjective and discursive influences which power – here understood to be hegemonic *male* power – maintains over appreciations of the respective marginality implied by disability or homosexuality. Alternatively, an apparently obvious but often overlooked fact can be reiterated: gay-disabled men are simultaneously hegemonic *and* marginalised subjects who cannot therefore be usefully characterised solely or even primarily according to their embodied convergence of disability and homosexuality. The contemporary gay-disabled male is, rather, an amalgam of past *and* present discourses and discursive practices relating to masculinity among which apparently radical contemporary frameworks may constitute just one element.[21] Indeed, the simultaneously retrospective and progressive, interrelated and cumulative elements of gay-disabled masculinity and experience is the aspect of this subject-position with which this analysis is perhaps most concerned. Thus, for instance, the gender ideologies and performative emphases with which the family is strongly allied should not be considered in isolation. Rather, they are held to be integrated into the discursive matrix which guides understandings of the inherent able-bodiedness of the exemplary and productive male subject as construed by capitalist socio-economic structures and relations. This is to suggest, and not without interpretative implications, that the aggregated gay-disabled male subject arises in consciousness as a distinctly ambiguous construct which is maintained as a *simultaneously* normative and pathologised (differentiated) entity. Or, that such males operate according to discernibly contrasting interior and exterior understandings of the ways in which they might access and/or utilise power based upon their dual potentiality as both hegemonic *and* marginalised subjects.

Under these conditions, gay-disabled marginality emerges as an equivalently ambiguous sensibility *and* discursive articulation of the ways in which non-hegemonic males are understood by themselves and others to be maintained in relation to power. Notwithstanding that their physical or emotional vulnerability to the activities and responses of hegemonic males may provide them with the basis of a critique of hetero-normative masculinity, other aspects of gay-disabled male experience imply more complex forms of subjective engagement with the dominant male gender construct. The details of gay-disabled experience suggest that the relations which exist between ostensibly hegemonic and marginalised masculinities cannot easily or even generally be characterised according to any simple domination-subordination dichotomy. Rather, the tensions between gay-disabled men's critique of hegemonic masculinities and their simultaneous propensity to emulate it emerge as a potentially confounding aspect of their accounts. Thus, and not least as the result of their frequent complicity with hegemonic male power as well as their validation of both its subjective and performative elements, male marginality emerges as a complex of understandings and experience which defies its easy characterisation.

Under all circumstances, gay-disabled men exhibit a subjectively organising concern with the authentic performance and experience of masculinity. Issues of disclosure, awareness of the always-present potential of violent regulation, attempts to 'pass' as straight males, and the hierarchisation of impairment according to its 'distance' from exemplary male physicality are dimensions of the constituted subjective aspiration to consider oneself, and to be viewed by others, as an ostensibly 'authentic' and unconflicted male. Moreover, and crucially, these dispositions again suggest that so far as multiply-differentiated men are concerned, power is most usefully conceptualised as a way of acting upon the acting subject so that forms of selfhood and subjectivity are not only maintained through physical restraint and coercion but through self-surveillance and self-correction to masculine norms.[22]

five

'I didn't have to go to a finishing school to learn how to be gay': Maori gay men's understandings of cultural and sexual identity

CLIVE ASPIN

Within a contemporary context, increasing numbers of Maori gay men are attaching significance to the term 'takatapui' (intimate friend of the same sex) as a culturally appropriate means of defining their sexual and cultural identity. The term is gaining renewed usage because of a number of factors, including a changing socio-political climate, a resurgence in the recognition of indigenous issues, gay community development and an increased recognition of cultural diversity within society. Of particular significance is the fact that these developments have occurred during a time of epidemic and, therefore, it is important to recognise the impact that HIV has had on Maori gay men's efforts to forge a uniquely specific identity that draws from the past as well as the present.

This chapter sets out to describe some elements of Maori gay masculinity as it is lived and experienced within contemporary society. The observations made here are derived from two principal sources: a nationwide survey of New Zealand men, and a series of interviews that I conducted with a number of Maori men. The survey took place in 1996 and the interviews took place in 1997 and 1998. Drawing on a limited number of sources, the discussion that follows attempts to describe some of the elements of pre-European Maori sexuality as they relate to gay sexuality within contemporary society. I then consider some of the ways in which these historical concepts have influenced how Maori gay men today perceive and describe their sexual and cultural identity. As well, I point to some of the other influences that have had an impact on how Maori gay men today express their masculinity, both as members of their whanau, hapu and iwi and of the wider community. These include influences derived from Western notions of sexuality that have developed and prevailed over the last two hundred years, gay community development in the latter part of the twentieth century, migration, and the impact of the HIV/AIDS epidemic.

Drawing from the past

Throughout the world, many aspects of indigenous societies have been heavily shaped, modified and even suppressed by the forces of colonising powers. For Maori this has meant that valued components of culture have been distorted or permanently lost. In the area of sexuality, the little information that remains about sexuality in pre-European Maori society comes from oral accounts and a few written documents dating from the time of first contact between Maori and non-Maori.

For example, we can be fairly sure that same-sex relations were sanctioned within Maori society. Support for such a claim comes from written evidence, oral accounts, as well as the knowledge that same-sex relations existed in other indigenous societies. The *Williams Dictionary of the Maori Language,*[1] first published in 1834, is an important record of Maori society at the time of early contact between Maori and Europeans. It contains an entry that seems to provide concrete evidence of the existence of intimate same-sex relationships within traditional Maori society. While it is important to acknowledge that the term does not equate to the terms homosexual or gay as we understand them today, it does nevertheless suggest that such relationships did exist and that they were fully accepted within Maori society. The entry is the word 'takatapui', and it is supported by the following illustration:

> Ka moea taku tuakana e toku hoa takatapui.
> [My older sibling slept with my close friend (of the same sex)].

Of note here is that the person speaking is male and that he refers to his close male friend as 'takatapui'. The takatapui is Tiki, the close and intimate male friend of Tutanekai. The story of Tutanekai that has been passed down to present generations focuses purely on the relationship between Tutanekai and his beautiful princess, Hinemoa. As with many similar stories from our past, this one too has been sanitised for a heterosexual audience to the extent that the other strand of Tutanekai's friendships has been downplayed or overlooked. In an effort to portray a solely heterosexual hero, anything that suggested the existence of homosexuality was suppressed.

Informing the present

Contemporary indigenous forms of identity have been constructed in relation to colonialism and, invariably, are based on measures designed to retain traditional concepts of the world. Within the Pacific, this has meant that minority indigenous cultures have struggled to assert themselves in relation to dominant majority cultures.[2] In relation to sexual identity, this mix of resistance and assertion has led to the development of concepts of sexuality that are unique to a contemporary context while still retaining important links with past expressions of sexuality.

In New Zealand, takatapui identity is an attempt to reconcile the present with the past. The word has recently been embraced by gay men, lesbian women and transgendered people who also identify as Maori, as a culturally appropriate term to define their sexualities. The full meaning of the term is best understood in relation to its historical and more recent usages.

In general, we can be sure that sexual expression in pre-European Maori society was somewhat different from what it is today. The processes of colonisation and religion have had a profound effect on the ways in which Maori express their sexuality within contemporary New Zealand. The imposition of the colonialists' view of sexuality has meant that traditional views and understandings of Maori sexuality have become blurred, misinterpreted or lost completely.

Evidence that remains today concerning traditional forms of sexual expression is derived from oral accounts as well as some few written documents. The arrival of missionaries meant that the oral tradition was broken and that some aspects of sexuality were omitted from the repertoire of information that was passed on. Moreover, the missionaries and early commentators set about recording Maori society through Victorian eyes, taking particular care to omit those features which might cause offence. In his detailed account of precolonial indigenous expressions of sexuality, the contemporary commentator Bleys provides ample evidence of the ways in which European commentators interpreted indigenous cultures according to existing Western paradigms.[3] He refers to 'the mixture of fascination and horror' that early writers brought to their accounts of indigenous societies. In their quest to discover the human race in an untarnished state, European voyagers were unsure about how to describe the variety of sexual expression that they encountered. Bleys cites cross-gender roles in America as particularly problematic as a result of the fact that similar cases were unknown in the countries from which commentators came. In the case of cross-gender roles in American Indian societies, for example, commentators encountered difficulties in describing men who exhibited behaviour and social roles associated with women. Furthermore, commentators tended to associate this perceived female behaviour with passivity in sexual relations and ultimately the abominable 'sin' of sodomy.

There have been numerous examples throughout history of colonisers applying Western paradigms to describe the sexual practice of colonised people. In the US, for example, all cross-gender roles were described by one blanket term such as *berdache*. *Berdache* was used to describe homosexual orientation. The term comes from the Middle East where it was used to describe a catamite or male sex slave, and was first used in North America by French fur traders who applied the term to anyone who practised receptive anal intercourse.[4] As Tafoya points out, such usage was inappropriate and ignored the existence of more than two hundred Native American tribes, each with its own distinct language and culture. Many of these languages had their own culturally specific terms to describe different forms of sexual orientation. Tafoya cites *nadleeh* (Navajo), *bote* (Crow) and *winkte* (Lakota) as examples of terms that denote multiple genders in their particular languages and traditions and, as a result, cannot be encapsulated in a single term such as *berdache*. In her commentary on the use of the term in a contemporary context, Jacobs describes how non-Native people embraced the term enthusiastically in their efforts to find historical equivalents to contemporary expressions of homosexuality.[5] While these efforts may have suited the purposes of those on the outside of the Native American community, they did nothing to alleviate the discrimination to which Native American gay, lesbian, transgendered people or two-spirit people have been subjected since colonisation.

In a similar manner, the actual nature and variety of sexual expression throughout the world has been suppressed or obliterated by the imposition of Western paradigms on colonised societies. In fact, as Bleys has argued, sexuality has been used as a means of proving that colonised people were inferior and in need of the superior wisdom of the coloniser:

> Sexuality thus became a vehicle of propaganda not only against the paganism of indigenous populations, but also against their presumed cultural inferiority. Sodomy, though common only in very particular circumstances and pursued by only a small group of the entire population, would be represented accordingly as ubiquitous, thus justifying its suppression through military and political violence.[6]

This imposition of a narrow view of sexuality must be seen as part of a wider picture whereby the world was divided according to a system of binaries based on 'them' and 'us'. This limited view of the world has had a profound effect on the way in which people today frame their sense of self-identity, as explained by Said:

> The construction of identity … involves establishing opposites and 'others' whose actuality is always subject to the continuous interpretation and re-interpretation of their differences from 'us.' Each age and society re-creates its 'Others'. Far from a static thing then, identity of self and of 'other' is a much worked-over historical, social, intellectual, and political process that takes place as a contest involving individuals and institutions in all societies.[7]

An understanding of the historical and social construction of sexuality in minority cultures helps to explain why traditional concepts of sexuality have been blurred over time. In the Pacific region, for example, colonisation has had a profound effect on contemporary forms of sexual expression. Until the arrival of colonial forces, the peoples of the Pacific enjoyed and shared a worldview in which sexuality in its many forms played a fundamental role in shaping the social structure of the region. Kahaleole Chang Hall and Kauanui have described the effects of the imposition of colonialist paradigms on Pacific peoples:

> The discrete analytical categories of 'homosexuality', and more fundamentally 'sexuality' itself, are a colonial imposition which only address the realities of a small part of the spectrum of Pacific people who have sexual and love relationships with members of their own sex. It also mistakenly thrusts those who transgress strict Western gender boundaries, but not sexual boundaries into this narrow conception of sexuality.[8]

Historical expressions of sexuality

In New Zealand, contemporary commentators on Maori sexuality have referred to some of the factors that marked traditional Maori sexual expression as different from the forms of sexual expression that are sanctioned within a contemporary context. Ngahuia Te Awekotoku, in her commentary on traditional Maori society, has asserted, 'Sexuality was enjoyed in many forms. People chose partners of either sex for pleasure, and same-sex love was not condemned or vilified'.[9] In reference to homosexuality, she has stated:

> Over the decades of colonisation the homosexual, and more certainly the lesbian, became invisible. Little is known of homosexuality as it occurred in traditional Maori society. My informants unanimously assure me that the incidence of it, both male and female, was marked.[10]

Timoti Karetu, in his keynote speech at the hui on Maori Reproductive Health and HIV/AIDS, reminded us of the central role that was given to sexuality in day-to-day life.[11] As shown in whakapapa, it was not uncommon for some ancestors to have multiple sexual partners, with this being viewed as a source of pride rather than condemnation. Moreover, people were not condemned because of sexual behaviour or sexual persuasion. It is worth emphasising that a broad and varied range of sexual expression is likely to have been fully supported and sanctioned at all levels of Maori society, at whose core lie whanau, hapu and iwi.

Contemporary expressions of sexuality

Members of sexual minorities within contemporary Maori society draw considerable strength and inspiration from the knowledge that the word takatapui existed within pre-European Maori society. Today, there are clear signs that the word is being reclaimed and used within a contemporary context. The brief discussion that follows traces the usage of the term within the last decade.

In 1992, a small number of men in Auckland established a support group for Maori gay men and chose the title 'Te Waka Awhina Tane' to describe themselves. The group was formed to provide support for Maori gay men who felt ostracised within the gay community. One of its founders explained his motivation for helping to establish the group:

> When I was coming out in the late 1980s early 90s we could celebrate our gayness but we couldn't celebrate our Maoriness within the gay, the prescribed gay culture

> then, so we created our own group, our own space, our own safe space culturally and sexually.[12]

A feature of the group was that members used the term takatapui to describe their sexuality. In their report to the Public Health Commission on the health needs of Maori gay men, Herewini and Sheridan explained the meanings behind the use of the term takatapui:

> The phrase *Takatapui Tane Maori* is preferred by some Maori homosexual men in the Tamaki Makau Rau/Auckland area as the appropriate terminology by which to identify themselves. *Takatapui Tane Maori* is understood by the authors of this report to include Maori males who identify as gay, bisexual or transgender, or who have sex with other males, or who by orientation are physically attracted to other males. It is therefore broader in scope than the phrase Maori gay men but clearly includes the latter.[13]

Soon after the establishment of Te Waka Awhina Takatapui it became apparent that other Maori within the gay community faced similar challenges to those experienced by Maori gay men. As a result, the brief of the original group was widened to embrace women as well as men. Today, as noted above, takatapui is used as a term to describe gay men, lesbians, bisexuals and transgendered people who also identify as Maori.

Multiple identities and their claims

An historical legacy of homophobia and discrimination has meant that within contemporary society men from minority cultural backgrounds who have sex with other men are often obliged to reconcile the multiple allegiances that dominate their lives. For those who identify as gay, bisexual or transsexual, efforts to acknowledge their sexuality must often be balanced with their commitments to their cultural communities. At times, efforts must be made to separate the two, ensuring that they do not overlap. Often these men need to be assisted to find ways of reconciling the multiple layers of their identity. Providing men with strategies to acknowledge their multiple layers of identity is particularly important in relation to access to health services, especially to HIV/AIDS information.

Prioritising one identity over another

Often men are obliged to acknowledge one aspect of their identity at the expense of another. As Gutierrez argues, non-heterosexual men need to be able to acknowledge all aspects of their identity in order to assume their rightful place in society alongside their heterosexual peers:

> Integration of our cultural, ethnic, sexual and geographic communities allows us to define our own lives and claim our rights to effective AIDS education and treatment, safety from hate crimes, and the opportunity to pursue a free and open social life.[14]

Initiatives which provide ways for men to acknowledge all dimensions of their identity can go some way towards improving self-esteem and, as a consequence, the health status of men from minority backgrounds. One successful example in New Zealand is that which relates to takatapui tane.

Takatapui identity

In their commentary on homosexually active men from ethnic minorities, Icard *et al.* make the point that men from ethnic minorities may experience difficulties in accommodating their multiple identities in their daily lives. Such men may experience competing allegiances which force them to give priority to one identity in favour of all others.

In a multi-cultural society like our own, communities often compete for the allegiance of members. In terms of the discussion in this chapter, homosexually active men of colour may feel the pull between their allegiances to a racial and ethnic community and their involvement in the gay community. There are two ways men of colour can handle the issue of community; that is, they may decide that they are gay or that they are a member of an ethnic minority, but not both. Conversely, they may attempt to piece together a 'multiple identity' – that is, an identity that integrates aspects of both groups.[15]

The discussion that follows describes a small group of gay men who have successfully pursued the latter strategy. It is based on the data from the interviews I conducted with the men. All respondents claimed both takatapui and gay identities. Names have been changed and personal identifying information has been omitted in order to ensure the men's anonymity.

The mean age of these men was thirty-two. While the numbers are too small to make any statistical comparison, this is in line with one of the findings of the *Male Call/Waea Mai, Tane Ma* report of Maori men who have sex with men.[16] Of the 170 Maori men who responded to *Male Call/Waea Mai, Tane Ma*, 53 (31.1 per cent of all Maori respondents) identified as takatapui, these men, on average, being younger than those who did not claim takatapui identity.

These younger men confirmed the fact that the term takatapui is enjoying renewed usage within a contemporary context. Three of them commented on the fact that it was not in use when they first came out. Consequently, each was able to identify the time when he had first claimed takatapui identity. Manu, who first came out as a teenager almost ten years ago, pointed out that he did not know about the term then. Now he regularly attends a takatapui hui and uses the term to describe his sexual identity:

> The word takatapui wasn't around when, if we're talking language, wasn't around when I was coming out so that it just, I don't know, it's a term that I have used to describe who I, you know who I am.

Neil explained that he knew about the term but has only applied it to himself over the last four years. Before this time he used other terms to describe his sexual identity. Such a process confirms the point that, for many people, sexual identity is fluid and changeable.[17]

Interviewer And how long have you called yourself takatapui?

Neil Ah, four years I would have claimed to be takatapui, prior to that I was gay (*laughter*) prior to that I was bi. Yeah. So, now it's … if anybody asks me what my sexual identity is I say well it's takatapui.

Interviewer And what made you make that transition four years ago?

Neil Well four years ago I basically met up with other takatapui that identified with it. I actually came across the term quite a while back – um, Ngahuia Te Awekotuku brought it up but it didn't sink in. I knew what she was talking about and I could identify with it.

Here Neil indicates the importance of context in helping him to arrive at an understanding of takatapui identity and its relevance for him. A similar situation was apparent for Mike who credited a recent takatapui hui as providing the motivation for his decision to claim takatapui identity.

Interviewer How do you describe your sexual identity?

Mike Now I describe it as takatapui tane, gay male.

Interviewer And how come you say that now?

Mike After being at this hui and identifying what takatapui is all about, and I feel more part of identifying as takatapui then as gay … just being in touch with takatapui, just being around the whole environment and the whole sharing and the learning you know … it gives me a deeper sense of being Maori, especially more so on the marae too.

Mike's experience is a clear example of how context provides a rationale for claiming takatapui identity. He was interviewed at a takatapui hui during which he came to claim takatapui identity as his preferred form of sexual identity. After attending this hui he no longer saw any conflict between his sexual and his cultural identity. As he sees it, the term takatapui allows the two important strands of his identity to be fully integrated within his sense of self.

Being able to identify as takatapui meant that he was able to identify more strongly as Maori ('It gives me a deeper sense of being Maori'). In particular, this allowed him to feel more comfortable about his participation in marae activities, something about which he has felt diffident in the past. Surely this is an example of how a complete sense of self-identity has benefits not only for the individual but also for the whanau, hapu and iwi. An individual Maori man with a complete sense of his sexual and cultural identity has more of a contribution to make to iwi activities than has a person with a compromised sense of self-identity.

Mike's comments on the takatapui hui bring into focus the importance of peers in helping one to arrive at an understanding of identity and its meanings.

Mike attached considerable importance to the fact that he had met other people who identified as *takatapui*. In the process he was able to comprehend the significance of belonging to a group of people with similar concerns and ideals. Weeks confirms that such events are important steps in the process of identity formation:

> Categorisations and self-categorisations, that is the process of identity formation may control, restrict and inhibit but simultaneously they provide 'comfort, security and assuredness'. And the precondition in turn for this has been a sense of wider ties, of what we can best call sexual community. It is in social relations that individual feelings become meaningful, and 'identity' possible.[18]

Mike also talked about the importance of his circle of friends when he lived for a time outside New Zealand. He described them as his social support group and identified common Polynesian ethnicity as their overriding link. He credited this group with giving him the support he needed when he was adapting to the difficulties of living in a new city and environment. It is noteworthy that no such support group was available when he went further away to live in the US. During this time he met a man with whom he had unprotected anal sex. He identified this as the time when he became infected with HIV.

RECLAIMING TAKATAPUI IDENTITY

In contrast to Mike, who had recently begun identifying as takatapui, four of the other men had claimed takatapui identity for a number of years. These respondents werc forthright about their choice of takatapui identity and its meaning in their lives.

Robert's discussion of takatapui identity illustrates clearly the role that such a description plays in his life as an individual and as a member of his whanau, hapu and iwi. He had no hesitation in declaring that he claimed takatapui identity. After stating that he was takatapui tane, he provided a concise translation of the phrase: 'a Maori gay man'. He made it obvious that his identity as takatapui was fundamental to his life and that it had a profound influence on his pattern of thinking.

> *Interviewer* How do you describe your sexual identity?
> *Robert* As takatapui tane, as a Maori gay man.
> *Interviewer* And to what extent is this identity important to you?
> *Robert* I think it's incredibly important to me. I think it's one of the things that forms a lot of my life and a lot of the ways in which I think.

For Maori who identify as takatapui, the cultural and sexual strands of identity are inseparable. Robert made this point clear when he outlined the effects that claiming takatapui identity had in his life.

> For myself it [takatapui identity] places me in a place of power. I feel that I have

> throughout the process of life and the things that I've been through, it's sort of like this thing of mana – almost this mana and being takatapui is one of the pous you know, it's a really important pou in my life. And with support of that and the history of it – whether or not it's been clouded by other people and whether or not the process of colonisation has clouded it for others within Maoridom – I still … I walk, with a pride about it; and I look, and I'm always really aware of that process of colonisation over the last 150 years and what that means for us as takatapui, and how it is incredibly important that we operate in a really proactive and positive manner.

Using himself as an example, Robert makes a number of important points about takatapui identity as it is lived within contemporary New Zealand. While his commentary refers to the use of takatapui identity within a contemporary context, he draws upon historical precedents to give meaning to the term. He recognises that the term derives from a legitimate historical context, a factor which contributes to the enhanced status of the term as a way of describing Maori sexuality today. He reminds us also that the process of colonisation has clouded the historical meaning of the term, and that takatapui today have a responsibility to reclaim that full meaning. He posits himself as an example of a contemporary Maori man who has taken steps to ensure that the term enters the language that is used to describe sexuality now and in the twenty-first century. Through the process of reclaiming a term that was formerly sanctioned by Maori society, he is now able to stand proud as a member of his whanau, hapu and iwi.

Arriving at takatapui identity

All the men I spoke to who claimed takatapui identity said that they had faced and overcome serious challenges in their lives. Manu had been dependent on non-prescription drugs and alcohol. When he lived overseas, he was unemployed and used sex as currency to make ends meet. Neil spent some years attempting to deny his Maori identity. He also did sex work and abused non-prescription drugs and alcohol. Robert left New Zealand and his family in order to come to terms with his sexuality. While living overseas he was bashed on several occasions. Te Ariki moved to Australia where he did sex work and was physically and verbally assaulted on more than one occasion. Mike became infected with HIV while he was overseas and his greatest challenge in recent times has been coming to terms with his status as an HIV positive man.

Today all of these men have been reintegrated into their whanau networks and, at the time that I spoke to them, they were holding down productive and fulfilling employment. All said that they now experienced far greater acceptance from their whanau than in the past. All of them made significant contributions to the whanau, hapu and iwi to which they belonged.

'They know what I've had to go through to get to where I'm at now': Overcoming challenges

It is worth tracing the path that has been followed by one of these respondents in order to understand the positive impact that a culturally appropriate identity can have on one's life. Manu left school at a young age and soon developed a drug and alcohol dependency which lasted until his early twenties. He sought professional help but this was unsuccessful. As he explains, counsellors focused on his dependency without exploring other issues in his life.

> I ended up as an out patient for like, over a period of a year in a psych unit. I, my parents had, well they kind of provided me with private alcohol and drug counselling and that was for a year but the issues, it took them a year to realise that the issue wasn't really around alcohol and drugs it was deeper than that, like they weren't actually very good therapists to tell you the truth because they couldn't deal with the sexuality component of my alcohol and drug abuse so ultimately I decided to come off this kind of therapy and it wasn't, it was purely A and D related that they didn't know what they were talking about and I did and my parents sent me over to Australia which is the first time I went to Australia to my aunty in Melbourne.

Living outside New Zealand exacerbated the problem. His dependency intensified. He was unable to find employment. Here he describes the extent of his drug use:

> I'd use drugs every day over there because I was unemployed, but mainly speed or coke so it, if we were going out we'd have ecstasy, a bag of speed and coke, but during the day it was generally speed or marijuana or alcohol, but it was on a daily basis.

The one currency that he was able to trade with was sex. Consequently, for the duration of his time there, he lived off his wits, his good looks and the kindness of others. Decisions about his life were made by others and he felt he had little option but to comply. Understandably, this posed serious risks to his health and well-being. Manu described several occasions when his life was at risk. He was severely bashed on more than one occasion. He was ejected from commercial venues. And his sexual practice often involved unprotected anal sex, something over which he felt he had no say.

Manu	I had lots of unprotected anal sex in Sydney and it didn't really matter who it was with.
Interviewer	Was that through choice or was it someone else's decision?
Manu	It was other people's decisions, I thought that that's what was expected of me basically so I mean I let it happen but I thought that that's what had to happen.

When I interviewed Manu, he had clearly regained control of his life. He was no longer dependent on drugs and alcohol. He was employed as a professional within a service organisation. He had been living in a monogamous relationship with his partner for some years. Both men played an active role in local takatapui activities. Manu felt that he and his partner provided positive role models for other young Maori who were facing challenges in their lives, especially ones related to their sexuality. And moreover both he and his partner were fully integrated into their whanau network, where both played important roles within their hapu and iwi. He located himself firmly within the family context, with his sexuality being a recognised and accepted component of his place within the family network.

> Our family unit, it's close, extended family the whole works, it's incredibly close so if someone was to insult me my mother would take that on board you know that would, wouldn't only be insulting me, it would be insulting my whole family and you just don't want to do that, cos they all wear it you know, they wear my, if I did something if I've got, if I shamed them then they all have to carry that as well but my sexuality does not shame them so they wear that with pride because they know what I've had to go through to get to where I'm at now all the struggle that I've had with my sexuality through being dependent on drugs and other things to where I am successfully living as a Maori or takatapui within a relationship independently.

Effects of takatapui identity on behaviour and health status

Unlike some of the other Maori men I have spoken to during the course of my research into sexual identity and sexual practice, takatapui respondents indicated that they were well integrated into their whanau, hapu and iwi networks. Claiming takatapui identity meant that they were able to look to their cultural heritage to facilitate this process of whanau reintegration. As McCarthy points out, an awareness of one's place within the whanau is essential to good health and well-being.[19] This applies all to whanau members, regardless of their age. Such a structure allows individual members the opportunity to explore and know their genealogy and history. From this knowledge derives an understanding of one's culture and ideally, an understanding of one's language. In the case of these men, four were competent speakers of te reo Maori and the fifth, Mike, had resolved to intensify his efforts to learn Maori.

Evidence from *Male Call/Waea Mai, Tane Ma* suggests that a minority of Maori gay men describe themselves as takatapui, and most live in one of New Zealand's larger urban areas. At the same time, however, it is likely that usage of this term will spread and the number of Maori men claiming takatapui identity will grow as networks of takatapui grow and develop. One person I spoke to during the course of my research emphasised the importance of takatapui networks in helping him to develop a strong sense of his own identity:

> I felt that I was a part of the Polynesian gay community, it was huge I mean it crossed all the, we were all united you know like we were takatapui no nga motu katoa you know it was from everywhere but with a, our common bond was that we had Polynesian blood in us and that's what kept us together you know, males, females, transgender, we all sort of stuck together and all supported each other, it was a really good circle.

It is likely that, over time, more and more Maori men will come to experience the solidarity that comes from belonging to a network that affirms one cultural and sexual identity and that this, in turn, will lead to greater numbers of men claiming takatapui identity as their preferred descriptor of their cultural and sexual identity.

Conclusion

It is clear that forms of sexual expression among indigenous people have developed in relation to a number of factors which include historical events as well as contemporary influences. In the case of Maori in New Zealand, historical factors such as colonisation and the imposition of Western paradigms have had a profound effect on how Maori view sexuality today. Contemporary influences include those which relate to religion, homophobia, whanau and attempts by institutions to control people's sexual lives.

This chapter has outlined some of the important features that have contributed to the development of takatapui identity within contemporary society. Sexuality within Maori society has, like sexuality in other cultural contexts, developed as a result of unique cultural and historical events. For Maori gay men in the contemporary world this has meant that notions of sexuality derive from Western concepts of sexuality which are common to gay men in other Western societies as well as traditional notions from pre-European Maori culture. Today, there is clear evidence that the term takatapui embraces both the Western and the traditional. An understanding of the complexities of sexuality is vital in understanding the ways in which Maori gay men order and structure their lives and this, in turn, is fundamental to designing effective sexual health promotion campaigns.

six

The Man with Two Brains: The Discursive Construction of the Unreasonable 'Penis-Self'

ANNIE POTTS

The centralisation of the penis in normative notions of heterosex may be interpreted as an effect of phallocentrism – that is, of the dominance of the phallus in Western cultural symbolism. In Lacanian theory the 'phallus' represents the Transcendental signified in the symbolic order (that is, the order of language and power). Power, authority, and control over desire are predicated on the subject's relation to the phallus.[1] The penis and the phallus are involved in a metonymical relationship, whereby the penis comes to represent the phallus, and thereby is invested with the power attributed to the phallus. By having a penis, men may seem closer to possessing the phallus and the power attributed to it. While much has been written on the metonymical association between the penis and the phallus,[2] this chapter focuses instead on the *synecdochical* relationship between the *penis* and the *man*. In particular, this relationship is explored with reference to the inside/outside dichotomy and the 'spatialisation' of sexed bodies.

Spatial tropes are pervasive in Western society. Indeed, Derrida argues that the inside/outside dichotomy is the 'matrix of all possible opposition'.[3] The modern human(ist) subject is constituted in terms of the spatial division, mind/body; this binary operates by crediting the mind with 'interiority': it resides 'inside', possesses the quality of 'depth', and is intimately aligned with the all-important 'self'. In contrast, the body occupies an inferior position on the 'outside' of 'personality', as a superficial, albeit necessary, shell or casing for the interior psyche. Furthermore, the spatialisation of subjectivity is gendered: mind – the 'superior' term in the hierarchical pairing – is associated with man, and body with woman. The differential spatialisation of subjectivity also produces specifically gendered 'experiences' of corporeality, depending on whether one's body is classified as female or male. However, in relation to *sexed bodies*, the inside/outside dichotomy is deployed in reverse: in this context, men are associated with exteriority (an effect of the visibility of the penis in a culture privileging visual over other sensory modalities) and women with interiority (due to their inner, invisible, reproductive organs).

Currently in feminist poststructuralist scholarship, conceptualisations of human subjectivity are being reworked to decentralise the mind/psyche through a 'reconfiguration of the body'.[4] This involves developing theories of human subjectivity which *include* corporeality, and which seek to destabilise those conventional philosophies which have, through their association with the binaries mind/body and inside/outside, arguably reproduced differential power relations between men and women. The term embodiment has become significant in feminist rewritings of subjectivity. It refers to '... the values, perceptions and gestures that are inscribed in and through the body and how we live these experiences through our bodies as men and women'.[5] Braidotti writes: 'The starting point for most feminist redefinitions of subjectivity is a new form of materialism, one that develops the notion of corporeal materiality by emphasising the embodied and therefore sexually differentiated structure of the speaking subject'.[6]

There are various theoretical paradigms which contribute to radical understandings of human subjectivity whereby the body is resituated. The model of the moebius strip is particularly useful for a reconceptualisation of the interrelation between corporeality and 'consciousness'.[7] This 'mathematical design' is defined by the *Collins English Dictionary* as 'a surface having only one side and one edge, formed by twisting one end of a rectangular strip through 180 degrees and joining it to the other end'.[8] The traditional representation of the human subject as split into separate territories of mind and body (inside and outside) is problematised by the moebius strip model, which shows how one 'region', through a process of torsion, becomes the other. Thus there is no clear boundary between inside and outside – no 'interior' corresponding to the mind, or 'exterior' of the body, for both/all are part of the same surface.[9]

Utilising the model of the moebius strip, this chapter explores the inscription of the dualism inside/outside on 'gendered' bodies: specifically, it is concerned with the signification and embodiment of hegemonic heterosexual male corporeality. However, while this study addresses the cultural production of certain 'corporealities', it does not merely involve a reversal of fortune for the 'physical' so that this becomes held in higher esteem than the 'mind'. Rather, it seeks to blur the once supposedly clear demarcations between mind and matter, exposing not only their inter-relatedness, but also the ambiguities and inconsistencies that mark representations of both. It focuses on the cultural production of hegemonic masculine bodies, explicating the ways in which the man perceives a split between his interior self and his exterior penis-self: a penis-self which is, in turn, granted an interiority – that has a mind of its own. It is argued that the exteriorisation of heterosexual male corporeality produces, and is reinforced by, the conflictive synecdochical relationship between the man and his penis, a relationship which is problematic from a safer sex perspective.

This chapter also uses extracts a feminist deconstructive analysis of extracts from interviews with Pakeha heterosexual men and women about male and female sexuality and heterosexual health.[10] Excerpts from academic articles and popular media items are also examined. There are obvious differences between these sources of investigative material (in terms of genre, social function, audience, and context, for example); however, because this investigation employs deconstructive analyses, these various 'texts' are examined in order to locate and analyse their discursive or rhetorical commonalities – that is, their common representational strategies. For instance, the excerpt from one of stand-up comedian Robin Williams's gags demonstrates how jokes about the penis *are* funny because they reflect shared assumptions about male sexuality in Western culture.

It is important to declare that the discursive examination here does not represent all men or, indeed, some essential characteristics of particular men. As Doreen Massey notes, such characteristics are 'traits of masculinity, not of men'.[11] Nevertheless, the strength of these depictions of 'normal' masculinity in Western culture suggests that many men will be 'pulled' towards them when 'understanding' or 'constructing' their sexual experiences.[12]

THE TRUTH IS *OUT THERE*: THE HIERARCHICAL SPATIALISATION OF SEXED BODIES

Luce Irigaray argues that '[Man's] sex (organ) presents itself as something external, through which he can love himself…'.[13] Indeed, it is the very *presence* of the penis – its 'self-evidence' in a culture which prioritises visual systems of representation – that guarantees the constitution of the 'sexed' male body as 'exterior' *and* superior: 'what can be seen (presence) is privileged over what cannot be seen (absence) and guarantees Being, hence the privilege of the penis which is elevated to the status of the Phallus'.[14]

The supposed superiority of the male body is endorsed by one of the female participants in the current study:

> Agnes — The first time I ever saw a … well, the first time I was ever with a boy or a man I was just absolutely *intrigued*. And then I realised that boys are sort of out there (gesturing outwards), like sort of they're all *out there* and I'm all in here (pointing inwards), and I mean really believing that boys outbeat us. Still do. I mean Bruce can go piss off the side of the boat and I can't, you know, I can't do that. Just anatomically I can't do that.

In this account of her visual introduction to penises, Agnes recalls that the first time she 'experienced' a penis, she 'experienced' a revelation: 'boys are sort of *out there* …. and I'm all in here'. This 'essential(ised)' sexual difference between men and women may be seen, however, to be the effect of the discursive spatialisation of 'sexed bodies': it demonstrates the differential territorialisation of body surfaces through the deployment of the inside/outside dichotomy and its superimposition on the dualism 'male/female'. In the construction of sexual/gendered – or carnal – subjectivities, the inside/outside dichotomy maps onto the hierarchical pairing of man/woman through a rotation which guarantees that man – whose association with 'mind' already grants him a superior *interiority* – maintains this privileged position through his body's construction as 'exterior'. Thus, the inside/outside opposition is capable of being deployed in different ways – even of being overturned – in the service of the pre-eminence of masculinity over femininity.[15] In contrast, the discursive constitution of woman's body as 'inside' positions her as inferior.

The symbolic advantage of male corporeal exteriority impacts in very material, and practical, ways on Agnes's view of men and women. She affirms the supremacy of male bodies: 'I mean really believing that boys outbeat us. Still do'. This is reduced to male anatomy – the penis – and its supposed advantage in urinating: the external position of the penis on the male body wins over the internal frustrations of the female body. Furthermore, the man in Agnes's narrative is urinating 'off the side of the boat', thus indicating a certain 'masculine' physical ease associated with 'the outdoors' – the external environment.[16]

However, the relationship between the man and his penis is complex: while the man's body may be envisaged as external to his self, the penis stands apart from the man. Often this leads to a battle of wills, in which the penis has a 'mind' of its own.

THIS INTELLIGENCE WHICH IS NOT ONE

> I don't simply have a penis: my penis is greater than itself[17]

Actor Robin Williams has this to say about men and their penises:

> Men, you know you have a tiny creature living between your legs that has no *memory* and no *conscience*. You know that. You know you have *no control*. There is no control over this tiny beast. You wake up in the morning, he's been up five minutes before you, like 'How you doing?' *No conscious control*. He's *there*! ... You have *no control*! It should be a separate creature. You should be able to take it off – boom! put him on the ground. Take him for a walk – he's got the rollers! ... That way you'd have some control! At least some control! Heel! Sit! You'd have some control then but as it is now you have *none*. No control at all ... We're *driven*! We're driven by this desire. By this *strange* creature. Wouldn't it be nice *sometimes* ... if you could go into a bar, buy him a drink once in a while. There'd be a big bar up here, a little bar down here for him. Go into the bar. Here, pull him out. He's looking up at you with his one good eye, like 'How you been, baby? Sorry about last night. I guess I got nervous. Fired off a couple of warning shots ... I am not an *animal*, I am a *sexual organ*!' It is this *creature*, this *lust*, but what compensates for this? There is also your heart – your heart is romance, going 'What about love?', 'What about poetry?', and he's down there going 'whatever works, babe, yeah'. Then above romance there's your mind going 'I believe you're both right. We must

> propagate the species but then we still must have conversation afterwards. That's why I'm looking for a woman who gives mind, if you catch my drift'. That's why we are driven to meet Miss Right. Or at least Miss Right Now … [18]

In Williams's portrayal, the penis is positioned not only *outside* of the male body, but also as a separate entity from the rest of him. At the same time it is a synecdoche for the male body: the external penis is granted interiority – consciousness, a mind (will) of its own. It has a life/ nature/ voice peculiar to this penis, divorced from the rational 'interiority' of the (male) mind. The penis thus becomes a miniature male person; hence, Williams portrays it as 'a tiny creature living between [men's] legs … It should be a separate creature'. This 'beast' talks to him; it apologises for its actions over which he (the man) has no control. This penis-person represents an homunculus parasitically attached to the man's body, simultaneously part of him and yet whose 'drives' are foreign or alien to him, and ultimately beyond his influence. The man is at the mercy of this penis-man, who, in Williams's account, possesses the personality of a naughty 'stud'. The comment 'I'm looking for a woman who gives mind' (gives head) enacts the moebius strip: what is sought is psychical and physical sex in one.

In the article 'Portrait of my Body', Phillip Lopate writes of his penis:

> This part of me, which is so synecdochically identified with the male body (as the term 'male member' indicates) has given me both too little, and too much, information about what it means to be a man. It has a personality like a cat. I have prayed to it to behave better, to be less frisky, or more; I have followed its nose in matters of love, ignoring good sense, and paid the price; but I have also come to appreciate that it has its own specialised form of intelligence which must be listened to, or another price will be extracted.[19]

Lopate's penis, perceived as feline, has a nose and a brain/mind whose form of intelligence is alien to the mind in the body to which the penis-cat is attached; moreover, this carnal intelligence commands attention from the man-body. The penis is thus positioned externally to the self. It remains outside the interiority of the mind, and is placed out of – away from – the exteriorised male body, although it inevitably contributes to this illusion of male bodies as exterior. (This is in contrast to the female body, which is always interior; even her 'cycles' continue to 'dominate' from the inside.) It appears as an out-pouch of the body's surface, but is invested with a depth of its own: a self external to the self (or perhaps man's 'external' self). Furthermore, while the penis stands in for, or up for, the man, the man may take the place of the penis, metaphorically speaking (hence the use of common vernacular terms such as 'stickman', 'dick' or 'prick', and phrases such as 'cocks on legs', to depict men in a derogatory way).

The popular notion of the penis as an entity in its own right is endorsed by women as well, albeit with some derision:

> *Interviewer* Do you think that there are differences between men's and women's sexualities?

Lilly	… I think that men will do anything or say anything to have sex. I mean I've – what I'm trying to say is that they're just –
Heather	Sluts. (*laughs*)
Lilly	Yeah and that their penises drive them … a lot of the time.
Heather	All the blood goes to their penis.
Lilly	Yeah and there's nothing left in their brain. (*Heather laughs*)

In this excerpt from a women's group discussion, Lilly and Heather imagine the blood flowing from the man's head in an expedition to the penis. Hence, the man no longer is able to think (except with his penis-brain). The penis then becomes the navigator – the 'driver' – of the man('s body).

The popular representation of male sexuality in terms of this penis/man split contributes to many men coming to understand their sexual bodies as dis-associated (as split-personalities), the rest of their bodies separated from their sexual penis-bodies. This phenomenon can be considered, in part, as a consequence of the binary division of mind/body. Here, mind represents the rational, superior interior of man, and body the inferior exterior 'vessel' for his mind. While invested with an internal consciousness of its own, the penis is still conceptualised as primarily a 'corporeal' entity, driven by 'primal' forces beyond the voice of reason, beyond the control of the male mind; thus man's external self-penis threatens his internal self-mind. Insofar as 'self-control, mastery of nature and of our nature, is a defining marker of the masculine state',[20] the potential chaos and intensity of the sexualised male body, under the control of the penis, represents a perceived disruption to masculine order and control.[21] Frosh argues:

> All this means that sex is both dangerously 'basic' and also somehow external – not p of what defines the man as 'man', as that advanced creature of rational mastery. Sex is always there, an obsession, but it is not part of us; being repudiated and repressed, it paradoxically threatens to take control … It represents a channel of personal 'truth', because it seems to contain the possibility of having intention, premeditation and self-consciousness overwhelmed by passion, yet it is disturbing for precisely that same reason – that the self, with its obsessionally embraced masculine armour, may be lost. Sexuality thus becomes relegated to the category of the bestial in man – rather like madness, perhaps – producing its characteristic response of fascination and fear.[22]

This construction allows men, in certain contexts, to experience their sexuality *more* physically,[23] particularly on occasions where the penis-'body (plus) mind' is perceived to overpower the male cerebral mind (and rational thought and behaviour). Arguably, it is the very demarcation between mind and body – which constructs men as having an external corporeal sexuality potentially beyond their rational 'reality' and control – which allows them to *experience* sex as a primarily corporeal phenomenon. Because sex for men is constituted as an externalised outwardly active feat, achieved at the expense of the mind and control – and thus separate from thought – it is understood as a bodily experience. In this scenario, the man, who now relinquishes control to his other person(ality), is, conveniently perhaps, removed from responsibility for his actions, which are, after all, the actions of his penis-body. This mode of 'reasoning' is frequently encountered in safer sex studies, where condom-use is problematised by participants as it interrupts the spontaneity demanded by the penis-body during sex.

Interviewer ... what sorts of things do you think might prevent or hinder a young heterosexual man from practising safe sex?

Toby ... I think there's little reason why if you haven't got a condom you *don't have* the sort of sex that will put you at risk. So far I've been able to live that out um but I'm sure for some people it might be difficult. They want to have sex. They have a drive to do it, and I've heard friends talk about it and there was certainly a friend of mine who grew up – her parents taught her 'don't touch a penis because once you *touch* it you'll let it *loose* and it just *won't be able to stop*'. See in that, there's that idea that once you start you can't stop, so that might be a reason. That's how people understand their sexuality.

In other contexts, this split between reason and passion operates by demanding men exert more control over their supposed animalistic urges.[24] In order to be more satisfying lovers, they are required to learn how to control mentally their sexual responses. It is in this context that the cerebral brain is deployed to overpower the penis-brain. Under such circumstances, men focus on 'performance' (or its associated anxieties). Any theory of hegemonic male sexuality must therefore take into account the complex negotiation – or altercation – between what is constructed as the male mind and what is constructed as the male body.

In the extract from Williams's show, the penis was construed as the driving force behind – the navigator of – the man's sexual body. However, this relationship appears to be symbiotic, for the male body also operates as a vehicle for the penis (the man's miniature male body). Moreover, the mini male-body, or penis-self, is a vehicle for his sperm (often popularly depicted as more diminutive versions of him). In accordance with prevalent masculinist perspectives in Western society, sperm are predominantly conceived of as active, mobile miniature 'beings' racing forth to achieve definite 'procreative' missions in accordance with heterosexualised biological imperatives.[25] In conventional heterosex, the emission and dispersion of sperm may be viewed as the final colonisation of the woman's body (the body of the other) by his; that is, the inside of his outside entering her inside, the final invasion of her body by the delegates of his. In this sense, ejaculation of sperm into the vagina represents his ability to continue penetrating her after penetration – hence the use of terms such as 'best swimmers' to depict sperm that survive to infiltrate her deepest recesses.

When the 'other brain engages': rationalising risky sexual behaviour

This valorising portrayal of the penis, in conjunction with the release of the miniature sperm-bodies that lodge within it, renders problematic certain heterosexual practices that may be safer in terms of preventing sexually transmitted diseases and unwanted pregnancies. For instance, the presence of a condom interferes with the passageway of the sperm: it sets up a border patrol through which the man's sperm bodies are not granted access. Indeed, when a condom is used, the sperm stay pretty much at home; they might make it out the gate, but are prohibited from venturing further. Most likely, they group around the door, a thwarted posse of conquistadors. The condom spells death to their military manoeuvres – military, because heterosexuality is discursively constructed in ways that associate masculine sexuality with violence. Whether it is the sperm 'piercing' the ovum, the penis penetrating the vagina, or the man sweeping the woman off her feet, her passive feminine sexuality succumbs to his active masculine sexuality, an active male sexuality that at times is 'seemingly' beyond his control. Or is it?

Interviewer Why isn't there some thought on the man's part of 'I need to protect myself', even if he's not going to think about protecting the partner, from what this person might have? It's sort of like a huge risk that they're taking.

Clarry I think women worry more, probably with good reason, but I mean I do think women spend more of their time worrying about their man's infidelity than vice versa and I think most men – well, we're *animals* like that, I mean we get sexy, you get a hard on, and your other brain engages, and I mean you just don't often – just don't – *you're not prepared to think* when you've got a hard on and you're trying to get into a woman like say for the first time … Most men … just think like, you know, a stiffie, got to have it, I'll deal with the possibility of AIDS later and of course there's those of us who know it's harder for men to catch – to get AIDS in conventional heterosexual sex than it is for women. What a hell of a rationale but I think we use it. I think I have in the past.

In this excerpt, male sexuality is construed as animalistic, out of the usual realm of male conscious control – 'we're *animals* like that, I mean we get sexy, you get a hard on, and your other brain engages … *you're not prepared to think* when you've got a hard on …'. The beastly penis which has reared its own head transmits its peculiarly sexually charged messages across the mind/body synapses to overrule rational cerebral thought, and override responsibility: it takes over from the man (who, after all, is his mind). But what thoughts might this 'other brain' generate? '… a stiffie, got to have it …': male reason is conquered – brainwashed – by his irrational, passionate other brain. In this version of masculinity, the body is externalised but it continues to be processed through the mind: hence, 'the man with two brains', one (penis)brain, which is focused on the corporeal world of sex, which has its own distinctly 'manly' intelligence and agendas, and which is detached from the masculine world of the other (cerebral)brain, which dominates conscious thought, memory, and reason.

In this construction, men are granted the best of both worlds: they possess an 'embodied consciousness'. In the case of both the penis-body and the male body, the body is an external envelope for an internal agency. Clarry uses the notion of a penis – his penis – with a mind/will of its own to distance himself from taking responsibility for ensuring safer sex is practised. It is the fault of this homuncular intelligence, this intelligence which is not one. However, when he says 'what a hell of a rationale but I think we use it', he inadvertently concedes that the depiction of the penis as a renegade miniature male body-with-mind-of-its-own is a mythical creation of his own mind (or in poststructuralist terms, a discursive construction). Men can thus deploy the mind/body split to their (supposed) advantage: the notion of the penis as a separate 'self' functions as an excuse for men who don't want to use condoms. This excuse operates both in advance and retroactively; for example, it provides the man with a justification for going ahead when anticipating sex ('gotta have it'), and thus permits him to regretfully excuse himself afterwards ('my other brain engaged').

Rather than simply replicating the inside/outside dichotomy, the penis is granted both exteriority (a position on the outside, distinct from the rest of the male body) and an interiority of its own. The penis's interiority functions as a form of corporeal intelligence, a twisting of the moebius strip; the distinction between body and mind becomes blurred. The male body has an interior – the mind – which is dominant over the inferior exterior body, but not the penis-body-plus-mind which operates according to its own principles (the 'reason' of passion).

The following extract, from an Australian television programme called *Sex, Guys and Videotape*, provides a further example of how the metaphorical construction of the penis as a miniature male person operates to produce a version of heterosexual masculine sexuality beyond the usual rationale and control attributed to the male mind. Elle McFeast is interviewing men about their experiences of being men and having sex:

Elle McFeast Have you ever been pressured into having sex or found yourself in the situation whereby you've had sex with someone but you haven't really wanted to?

Andrew Oh yeah, I have. That sounds like a real macho ego bullshit thing to say (*laughs*) but yeah, I have.

Elle Why did you go through with it? You just sort of felt like –

Andrew This is going to sound shocking (*men in background laugh*) but um on a couple of occasions, just cos I could. Cos it was there and it was just 'oh well why not?' That's how some – that's how a man's mind works every now and then. Just go 'oh well why not?'

Elle	Is that an example of your penis having a mind of its own?
Andrew	For sure. And as you get older hopefully you get more control and you go 'no, no, *think*', you know, you're at a pub or whatever, and you go 'no, no *think* of the repercussions. *Think* of how you're going to think after you've come', you know. I've got a – this is really very very graphic here but I've got a way of working out whether I really like a girl, and that is whether I'm with them or not with them, whether I'm by myself, if I think about them *immediately* after I've come, and if I *like* them immediately after when you're completely *asexual* for a few minutes – then you know you like them. If you don't, it's just a dick thing.[26]

To examine briefly this exchange, McFeast asked whether the men had ever felt a pressure to have sex, or whether they had actually had sex when they did not feel like it. Andrew admitted to having experienced a pressure on him to have sex; however, the form this 'coercion' revealed itself to take is very different from that experienced by women in heterosexual relations. Indeed, whether or not this 'pressure' may be classified as a demand from another person is debatable: what Andrew is alluding to is his obligation to respond to the appetite of his penis, his other self, his external self. Furthermore, because this 'compulsion' stems from his penis-person – his most masculine miniature male body (the embodiment of his maleness) – he is careful to resist any reference to this as a conscious willing action on his part, or rather as an intelligent (cerebral) choice. Moreover, while saying he has been pressured into sex by his penis, he does not construe this as a negative thing. Indeed this form of coercion takes on a decidedly positive quality, albeit one which must be modestly negotiated in front of his male peers: 'That sounds like a real macho ego bullshit thing to say … but yeah I have [been pressured]'. The penis has power over him: it is one up on him.

In contradiction to women's understandings of coercion in heterosexual relationships,[27] Andrew's coercive experience consists of *his 'taking advantage' of a situation where he could have sex*: 'This is going to sound shocking … but … on a couple of occasions, [I had sex] just cos I could. Cos it was there and it was just "oh well why not?" This is attributed to his penis having a psychology (mind and behaviour) of its own – 'that's how a man's mind works' – which Andrew hopes can be better 'controlled' as a man gets older, or matures. Thus, the penis is imparted with its particular penile developmental psychology: however, 'teaching' and 'disciplining' the penis is the job of the head/master, the man's cerebral brain, and unlike a child, the penis-person will always have to be supervised by the man-brain, for it will always be arrested in the genital stage.

Once the rational mind exerts some control over the penis-person, a man is able to 'think ahead' to the consequences of succumbing to the pressures of mindless (penis-minded) sex: '… you go, 'no, no, *think* of the repercussions.

Think of how you're going to *think* after you've come'. The male orgasm brings the man back to his 'real' interior mind from his other external 'sexual' mind of his penis-person. In this context, the intelligence of the penis is unreasonable; it is the antithesis of cerebral thought. Moreover, it is untruthful; an artificial intelligence, for the man can only determine his authentic feelings for his female partner in sex by noting whether he 'brings her to mind' after his penis-brain stops 'thinking'. This is accomplished during the recovery period following climax when the man is *'asexual'*; that is, when his penis, which after all *is* his sex, lies comatose. If he still thinks of her then, while his penis is temporarily uncomprehending, then he genuinely likes her. If not, 'it's just a dick thing'. Interestingly, as he can only come back to himself and thereby relate to others after his other self (penis) has had its way and been put to sleep, this begs the question: which 'self' is *prior*?

Conclusion

The inside/outside dichotomy produces disparately spatialised sexual subjectivities: for men, this manifests as an exteriorisation of their sexual-corporeality. Consequently, men tend to distance themselves from the behaviours of their bodies during sex. In this way, they may also exonerate themselves from responsibility in sexual matters. In a complex synecdochical relationship between man and penis – through the personification of the penis – the attitudes and behaviours of the penis-self are depicted as distinct from, and in opposition to, the conscious rational self-control of the man. This permits individual men to employ the penis-self as a disclaimer, in the flesh, for riskier heterosexual practices and heterosexual coercion. The discursive centralisation of the penis in male heterosexual pleasure also restricts the possibilities for other pleasurable and potentially safer sexual activities: it reduces the concept of 'real' heterosex to unfettered penile-vaginal penetration. This is problematic from a safer heterosex perspective, where condoms are culturally devalued for their supposed interference with the 'full' expression and sensation of the penis during penetrative sex. The predominance of the penis in notions of healthy and normal male sexuality also inhibits heterosexual men from 'thinking sexually' about/with other parts of their bodies, thereby preventing their discovery and enjoyment of diverse erotic experiences. This investigation indicates that sexual health promotion campaigns would benefit from the incorporation into such programmes of a critical understanding of the differential spatialisation of male and female bodies in Western culture. The study focused on hegemonic masculinity: future research might also examine the effect of the spatialisation of sexed corporealities on non-hegemonic male sexual subjectivities.[28]

seven

'Tits is Just an Accessory': Masculinity and Femininity in the Lives of Maori and Pacific Queens

HEATHER WORTH

> I really believed that I was a woman. Female. Even male, as well. So I didn't really have a problem with being male or female. So yeah, I was a boy … And people go – some of my queen friends go … why, why is it she just – be a woman or be a ... I said it's just – don't get hung up on that – society bullshit about being either or. You know? *(Louella)*[1]

> Modernism's crisis of legitimation, a crisis signalled in the term 'postmodernism', registers the faltering recognition that this complicious kinship of gendered binary divisions cannot be accepted complacently. If meaning is produced rather than simply given, then sexual identity, like any other identity, is a relational, processual entity that emerges through language and its peculiar economy. It follows from this that the hesitations that now interrupt orthodox accounts of truth and subjectivity have inevitably returned us to the perplexing questions of … identity.[2]

In her book *Gender Trouble: Feminism and the Subversion of Identity* Judith Butler postulates gender as performative: 'There is no gender identity behind the expressions of gender; that identity is performatively constituted by the very "expressions" that are said to be its results'.[3] Her central question is how the subject capitulates to the interpellation of power. She argues that subjectivity is possible only within subordination; subjectivity is tied to inescapable loss. Butler's particular interest is in how women come to have a 'passionate attachment' to their own subordination. Butler allows that gender cannot be summarily refused; but she also claims that taking up can never be strictly complied with; the subject and gender always carry within them ambivalence. This ambivalence, she argues, is played out through the parodic inhabiting of feminine normativity, an inhabiting which calls into question interpellation, because such a parody is 'a repetition of the law into hyperbole'.[4] Butler's further question is:

> What is meant by understanding gender as impersonation? Does this mean that one puts on a mask or persona, that there is a 'one' who precedes that 'putting on' who is something other than its gender from the start? Or does this miming, this

> impersonating precede and form the 'one' operating as its formative precondition rather than its dispensable artifice?'[5]

In the last chapter of *Gender Trouble*, and again in a chapter in *Bodies that Matter*, Butler utilises drag to make her point about this parodic constitution of gender. She argues that mimicry of 'the original' by drag queens 'reveals the fiction of gender because there is no original to parody, drag, [as a] ... reveals the original to be nothing other than a parody of the idea of the natural and original'.[6] Drag is not an extravagant replica of authentic or true femininity, but, like heterosexuality itself, a grandiose echo of the impossibility and the excess of gender.

In this chapter I take Butler's ideas of interpellation and drag and ask further questions. What kinds of interpellative calls do drag queens inhabit with regard to masculinity? Are drag queens gay or straight? How do Butler's ideas of ambivalence fit with notions of excess of gender? In order to provide some ways of thinking about these problems (if not providing answers to them) I will work through the potent empirical examples generated in the course of interviews with a group of ten South Auckland queens (six of whom were sex workers). These queens were part of a larger research project, *Frayed at the Margins: Underclass Men Who Have Sex With Men*, a study of the relationship between poverty and unsafe sex amongst men who have sex with men in South Auckland. Fenella, Lionel, Cherry, Louella, Helen, Jasmine, Pandora, Penny, Rhonda and Tara (all pseudonyms) described themselves as a combination of queen, *fa'afafine* (Samoan for 'the way of a woman'), woman, and/or girl. All of these ten subjects were either Maori or Pacific Island. Six had done or were still doing sex work, one as a male and a female, the others only as females.

Femininity

> '... your boy's going to be an auntie when he's older' *(Lionel, reporting a conversation between a cousin and his parents)*
>
> [I] used to go to, used to go to work in dresses even. Yeah ... I made it known to a lot of people, that I was very queer ... Yeah, well see, I don't care. Even now, I, I walk around, Miss Prancing around Manukau, and I don't care what people think.

Rivers of ink have been spilt on what really constitutes a drag queen. Most literature views queens as simply drawing upon stereotypes of femininity and using them as satire, rather than presenting realistic images of women. Most of the studies of queens examine how the drag queen highlights and parodies sex and gender differences by using 'her' male body as the framework on which exaggerated symbols of femininity are constructed and played out. Their attraction to other men and their feminine appearance and demeanour seem to position them in the realm of the feminine, outside that of the masculine; yet their biological constitution, by the standards of dominant society, places them in the realm of the masculine. But most importantly, queens do not 'merely elaborate a directly feminine image; there is an articulation and a refraction'.[7]

In this study that kind of excessive femininity was present. Many of the girls wore glamorous clothes to their interviews. As well, a number of the girls did drag shows. Being a successful performer is one way to counter the negative experiences often encountered by queens and *fa'afafine.* Many people in this study aspired to successful careers as performers, singers and dancers. This perhaps explains why some do sex work in order to be sufficiently prepared for their stage appearances (even if, as Helen and Penny describe, this sometimes results in a problematic dichotomy between 'show girl' and 'whore'). Penny says she uses her unemployment benefit to pay the rent and then the money she gets from sex work for her entertainment needs and to buy outfits for her (drag) show appearances: 'To be quite honest, to be really honest with myself, I'm still doing it now. Yeah, yeah, I'm a show girl'. There are also cultural resonances and continuities for the continued existence of a performing role for queens and *fa'afafine* in both Maori and Pacific Island societies.

But alongside the desire for glamour and performance there was also a desire to *be* a woman, and in some cases to *not be* a man. From an early age Penny had a real sense of unease with being a boy. 'Even back then, when I was at primary – I mean at intermediate, I felt like a real – I felt like I was a woman, trapped in a man's body'. Helen's fervent desire when she was at school was to be a girl:

> I remember when I was a lot younger, I always used to say my prayers in case I'd wake up in the morning and I've got long hair – and breasts, and one of those … I mean – wake up, oh it's still there! Damn it. Yeah, that was me in the mornings.

Jasmine is proud of her breasts: 'I have breasts. I like to grow my breasts like that – I'm the only one who has breasts'. When Fenella was asked what gender she called herself, she answered:

> I call myself … well before, before I moved here, I was ashamed to say something like I was a real girl, but now, I'm, I'm not ashamed of it. I mean, probably before I moved here too, because when I was staying in Massey and I wasn't ashamed to say I was a queen, or you know, because everybody knows.

She went on to explain: 'I consider myself as a hundred per cent female, and that's the way I live my life, every day'. Does this desire to 'pass' as a woman mean that these girls are no longer queens? All the girls in this study saw themselves as queens, as well as numerous other identities. Their identity as a queen is of course inflected with ethnicity. Several of the subjects in this study identified as *fa'afafine*, and a number of these queens called themselves *'fa'afafine'. Fa'afafine* are not, according to Besnier, 'representatives of femaleness as a coherent and unitary category, but rather they align themselves with *specific instantiations* of womanhood in various contexts'.[8] Besnier argues that the gender liminality in the contemporary Pacific 'is further complicated by the presence, particularly in the more acculturated areas of the region, of gay identities and perhaps communities that differ from "traditional" gender liminality and resemble patterns observable in Western contexts'.[9] Louella, whose words preface this chapter, is in her late twenties, is a New Zealand-born Samoan and calls herself *'fa'afafine'*:

> *Fa'afafine* means ... like a woman, so – that's broad as it says … And I'm quite comfortable like that. That's, that's where … that's how broad it is. It's very inclusive, it's not exclusive … *fa'afafine* is very broad. It means femininity to me. So everyone has femininity in them, so everyone's a *fa'afafine,* in one, some sense. *(Louella)*

But she is not *fa'afafine* in any 'traditional' sense. Like the other queens in our study, she carries with her Western notions of identity and difference, sex and gender. And the kinds of problematisations of *fa'afafine* at the turn of the millennium are those of femininity in late modernity.

The problematics of masculinity

> I'll always be Mum and Dad's son, you know. God, I mean I was born a – I'm born a man, I was born a man, you know? And ... but it ... it doesn't just end there, you know? I was born a man, but it doesn't make who I am. I mean I identify with possibly everything. And, you know, my, my female side and my masculine side … I'm totally my Dad's son. *(Rhonda)*

In the narrative above, Rhonda talks about herself as both girl and boy, as being a son to her father. If we worry about Butler's account of interpellation such that subjects are insistently this or that and continually account for themselves anew, doomed to reiterate gender in its most subjugating form, how then do we theorise Rhonda's 'strangeness' as both man and woman, or how do we comprehend what it means for Fenella to be a 'bad-ass honey with a difference'?

Identity, and its Ur-category, 'masculinity', is a central trope of late modernity. Much of the scholarship on masculinities describes and critiques a hierarchy in which Western heterosexual masculinity is phallocentrically read. Hegemonic masculinity has supremacy over femininity, and marginal masculinities and sexualities, particularly those of non-white men. Connell, for example, defines hegemonic masculinity as 'the configuration of gender practice which embodies the currently accepted answer to the problem of the legitimacy of patriarchy, which guarantees (or is taken to guarantee) the dominant position of men and the subordination of women'.[10]

Michel Foucault has argued that in the West we are 'dominated by the problem of the deep truth of the reality of our sex life'.[11] We have come to believe that the realisation and naming of the individual's 'true self' is intimately intertwined with sexuality. Masculinity remains primarily a gendered form with an accompanying 'erasure' of sexuality. But this disavowal of sexuality within the common sense usage of masculinity in effect means that masculinity is heterosexually marked. As well, Butler argues that 'proper' forms of masculinity almost inevitably imply a heterosexual identity:

> Homophobia often operates through the attribution of a damaged, failed, or otherwise abject gender to homosexuals, that is calling gay men 'feminine' or calling lesbians 'masculine,' and because the homophobic terror over performing homosexual acts, where it exists, is often also a terror over losing proper gender ('no longer being a real or proper man' or 'no longer being a real or proper woman').[12]

Four of the queens in our study also saw themselves as men. Louella sees herself as male and doesn't 'have a problem with being male or female'; Fenella argues, 'I was born a man', Helen knows she is a guy. However, in the lives of the queens of South Auckland who took part in the study, masculinity is anything but a stable hegemonic category. While most literature would argue that drag queens do not attempt an androgynous image and consciously exaggerate femininity, Louella seems an exception; masculinity sits beside femininity in a comfortable cohabitation. She puts it like this: "Some days I will go with tits, and some days I don't. I'll dress up like a woman and have fun, and then I'll pay respect to my masculinity and not put on a dress. And I feel really happy with that. Tits for me is an accessory'. In fact, I saw Louella with tits for the very first time a year after the interviews were carried out. In all my previous meetings with her she always dressed in 'boy' clothes, but with makeup and painted fingernails. She elucidates her position by arguing: 'We [should] look at not just gender, sexual … like trans-gender or whatever, [but] look at everybody – at how everyone has their own independent, individuality – and what – identity, of their own'. Helen spoke of the difficulties in this way:

> Sometimes there was, you know, you know, you know that you want to be a girl, but then you know that because you're a guy, you have these needs as well, so I guess, more or less, in a way.

Fenella's position is less strongly articulated, but she too states:

> I was born a man, but it doesn't make who I am. I mean I identify with possibly everything. And, you know, my, my female side and my masculine side …

Is drag straight or gay?

Interviewer: So now, you see, like, gay man as different from *fa'afafine*?

Respondent: Oh yeah. Yeah. Totally. Because … I'd go for a gay man, but I wouldn't go for a *fa'afafine*. Because *fa'afafine,* to me is … really, like, myself … I'd be, oh no, that's incest. Do you know what I mean? Yeah, so, when I talk about *fa'afafine*, it's like … yeah. You're a girl. Whereas there may be a guy, a gay male, and we're, oh yum, he's delicious, it's like that.

Is drag, as Butler has argued, a straight phenomenon? Is it about the stabilising of heterosexuality by allegorising 'the mundane and psychic and performative practices by which heterosexualised genders form themselves through the renunciation of the *possibility* of homosexuality'.[13] Things do not seem so simple for the queens in this study. A number of them saw themselves as gay. Helen stated, 'Yeah, I'm gay. Yeah, I'd say I am, I am ... I'm gay. But I'm, I'm not gay in, in a way where it's, it's wrong, you know. I don't feel it's wrong. I feel that ... being gay is another term for well, you're not heterosexual and you're not bi-sexual'. Pandora, on the other hand, saw herself as gay, but also considered the possibility of being straight:'[I'm] definitely gay. But ... maybe if I meet – the right female, in, in the future, it could change. Yeah. I've been with a female before'. Cherry, who classified herself as always having been a cross-dresser, argued: 'I'm just a gay male. I'm not – a transsexual, I'm not ... you know, I'm not any of the – female impersonating – oh well, I'm a cross-dresser. Yeah, that's how I class myself. Yeah'. Louella was asked:

Interviewer: You obviously don't think of yourself as a gay man. Can you just explain a little bit about that?

Louella: OK, a gay man to me, would be … well, yeah, I, I think I'm a gay man. Because I'm, male – biologically, gender – genitalia wise, I am male, so yeah, I am, I'm a gay male. But I'm also *fa'afafine* …

In the movie *To Wong Foo Love* Julie Newmar, the drag character Noxeema, declares, 'When a gay man has way too much fashion sense for one gender, he is a drag queen'. The sexual identity of the drag queen as gay male extends the challenge to paradigmatic sex and gender in which heterosexual identity is linked with masculinity and femininity.

Leon Pettiway, in his book *Honey, Honey, Miss Thang*, insists that his African-American drug-using, street-walking hustlers 'are gay men [who] dress and view themselves as women'.[14] Similarly Gary Dowsett's book, *Practicing Desire,* deals, in one chapter, with the connection between gayness and drag. In discussing one of his characters, a drag queen named Harriet, Dowsett rightly sums up the profound consequences for each person's assignment to one or other side of the man/woman binary. However, both Dowsett's and Pettiway's books are problematic in their view of drag through a lens of homosexuality. Thus, Harriet's biography is 'the historically constructed experience of living a gay life'.[15] This seems inadequate to the morphology of subjects like ours whose lives encompass both Western and Pacific cultures, and who see themselves as more than gay men.

As well, for some of our respondents, identifying as gay was not an option. Fenella's response was, 'I'm not a gay man in a dress'. Being called gay was 'confusing' and she believed that she was completely female:

> being a *fa'afafine*, what it means to me, or what it is to me, is that – I don't consider myself gay. Because to me, I consider myself as

a hundred percent female, and that's the way I live my life, every day. And … when – I've been called gay, when people call me gay, I look at myself and I go no, a gay man, I am [a] different thing.

Interviewer: Wearing girls'clothes, is that a different thing, then, or is it part of the same thing?

Fenella: Yeah, I, I … I think it is. Being gay and actually – being in, in a dress, and you know, sort of – switching gender roles. I think it's … it's not gay at all. I don't really think it's gay.

For Helen being gay was a 'stage' that she went through, on the way to some other gender/sexual identity:

> I consider myself as … really, I'm sort of halfway, just over – I'm just over the gay … Oh sorry, just past the gay stage – like, OK, you've got a line here, you've got your gay – you're gay part, sort of like me growing up. And then – I've just sort of slightly stepped over to the transsexual side.

The literature on drag, as the domain of either gay or straight men, and in both developed and underdeveloped countries, does not recognise queens as women, but rather as either men, or as a third gender group, or as people in-between genders. But in our study, many of the queens saw themselves as not a single gender group, but rather as having both genders or more than both. Their identities were multiple and shifting in time and space. They spoke about being male and/or female simultaneously and in seemingly contradictory ways about their present sex and gender during the interview. Often in the same sentence or two they changed from female to male pronouns and back again at will. It has therefore been a source of real consternation to know whether to call these respondents 'men' or 'women' or 'girls', 'he' or 'she', so caught are we in the Western sexualisation of language.

Take Fenella, for example:

> We have the female side, we've got the men's, the straight side of ... I don't know who I'd class myself … I like, I like to call myself a transsexual, but I know I'm not. I'm only fooling myself, but yeah, I don't know. Just as a human being, I guess. I'm just a human being.

Helen argues that she was born a man and that she will always be a son to her parents. But she understands that sexual and gender identity does not end at birth, that her identity 'as possibly everything', signals the paradox of gender and sexuality.

And Jasmine's story about her partner seeing her penis for the first time adds yet another dimension to the problematics of masculinity and femininity:

> I played a trick on him. Which is, to make him think how, how would he feel if I told him I was a man. And then he goes, where is your penis? And I showed it to him and he just couldn't believe it. Because we bath together, we have a shower together, and ... he never sees it, until the night I told him. And I showed it to him.

> Then he goes ... this is not real. But it was, you know, he just thought it was not real. He just thought it was one of those put-on penises you can put on and, you know, the vibrator or whatever you call it. Then I said, let me try it out for you, because I've always wanted to do this. I want to try with him. And then we tried it, and ... he, he's going ... this is not real, it doesn't feel real. And then I take it out and I just – hid it again. And then when he, when he went to have a shower, I didn't bring it out again, I just hid it. And then he goes see, you're not a, you're not a man, you're a woman. And this is the Jasmine I'm in love with. The girl. You know, not a man. But sometimes it just makes me wonder. How come he just couldn't tell. You know?

It is not enough to see Jasmine's boyfriend as disavowing the reality of her penis. It is more that Jasmine's penis, the very anatomy which ought to be the bedrock on which her sex is determined (if not her gender) has no meaning for him.

Ambivalent or excessive gender

> Identification is always an ambivalent process ... This 'being a man' and this 'being a woman' are internally unstable affairs. They are always beset by ambivalence precisely because there is a cost in every identification, the loss of some other set of identifications, the forcible approximation of a norm one never chooses, a norm that chooses us, but which we occupy reverse, resignify to the extent that the norm fails to determine us completely.[16]

> Yeah, I go out as a girl. And I know that sometimes I get sprung as a, as a boy, but it doesn't bother me. I think well hey, I'm who, I'm who I am. *(Helen)*

In the Western discourse of sexuality, 'Being' is sexually marked masculine, and masculinity is ascribed as prior to sexual difference.[17] The idea that identity is masculine dominates Western thought and is part of what Kirby calls 'the separation and privileging of the ideational over the material, male over female'.[18] But the narratives of the ten South Auckland queens described here attest to masculinity's contestability. They indicate the ways in which masculine identity is never hegemonic, in that it can be ruptured and broken. While their stories are a potent empirical example, I am not arguing that it is these queens' marginality and difference that allows for such a shattering to occur. Rather, that masculinity itself bears these characteristics as a foundational principle. Derrida's notion of *différance* is helpful here; identity, he argues, is produced through the differences of difference.[19] This production of difference (for this is what *différance* does), maintains identity. Thus one can posit that it is femininity that produces masculinity and vice versa; that rather than being two opposing forces on either side of the binary from one another, masculinity and femininity are integral to each other's identity:

> The breach in the identity and being of the sovereign subject ... is a constitutive breaching, a recalling and differentiating within the subject, which calls it into

presence ... This very breach opens identity to a force field of differences in which the binary divisions ... are impossibly implicated.[20]

Using Butler's terms, Cherry, Fenella, Helen, Jasmine, Lionel, Louella, Pandora, Penny, Rhonda and Tara are doing drag, they are 'imitating' femininity, and this process is an ambivalent one of being implicated in the regimes of power by which one is constituted. The interpellating calls and reiteration of the law in these queens' lived experience are, like those of heterosexual women, gay men and other gender identities, 'a constant and repeated effort to imitate [femininity's] own idealisations'.[21] In other words, there is an ideal of gender that none of us can ever fully embody.

But these queens are man *and* woman, masculine *and* feminine. In fact the very 'perversity' of their identity, both its determination and waywardness, seems not to be a mistake that can be corrected. We may just have to accept that interpellation never quite works.

Jacques Derrida has written in a number of essays about the legislative character of the subject and gender. He understands the law of gender to be that classificatory and enforceable principle of non-contamination and non-contradiction, of binary opposites man/woman. Derrida's essay 'The Law of Genre' questions not only literary genre but also genus (from whence we get notions such as generation), and gender (the French genre of course is the same word). He argues: '[A]s soon as genre announces itself, one must respect a norm, one must not cross a line of demarcation, one must not risk impurity, anomaly or monstrosity'.[22] But he also asserts that the law of subjectivity and gender can be refused; it always potentially exceeds the boundaries that bring it into being. By its very constitution the law of gender is constitutively unable to maintain absolute purity. This failing is generative – at the same time as it produces identity (gender) it disrupts it. Deconstruction, of course, has a fixation with identity and its peculiar capacity for differentiation.

The law demands two sexes: male, female; and that we choose between them (genres are *not* to be mixed). It also demands two or maybe three genders (masculine, feminine and perhaps transsexuals). And it also demands that we do not mix what Derrida calls 'the essential purity' of gender's identity. How does the Derridean problematic of genre (of gender difference and identity) fit with these *fa'afafines'* experiences? In the lives of these young queens and *fa'afafine* in South Auckland at the turn of the new millennium, this does not seem applicable. The law of genre does not seem to hold. They refuse such an edict, such an interdiction. Their genders are in excess of their genre, of the law of gender. In fact the very perversity of their gender, both its determination and waywardness, seems not a mistake that can be corrected. Derrida posits another possibility:

Suppose for a moment that it was impossible *not* to mix genres [my italics]. What if there were, lodged within the heart of the law itself, a law of impurity or a principle

> of contamination? And suppose the condition for the possibility of the law were the *a priori* of a counter-law, an axiom of impossibility that would confound its sense, order and reason.[23]

As we can see from the stories of these women, they disrupt the law by a spilling over of identity. It is not just that they cannot choose; more importantly and problematically, they want it all. It is not as if they are free-floating, unconnected to gender. It is their very engendering which marks them.

Speaking of his film *M Butterfly* in relation to Neil Jordan's *The Crying Game*, which was released when the former was in production, Cronenberg states: '*The Crying Game* made that thing of two men having a love affair – where one didn't know that the other one was a man – kind of sweet and innocent and pure and, in a weird way, not threatening … I think it's because she (Jaye Davidson) really is a woman, even though she's got a cock …' In this way the law, which is often figured as an interdiction, as the negativity of a boundary which cannot be crossed, becomes a process of double affirmation (a yes, yes to it all). Their excessive genders are not a call for an indeterminacy of identity, part of the West's obsession with the Other's exoticism, but a necessity born of the articulation of the femaleness of this morphology. If genre/genders pass into each other, it permits an engendering of *fa'afafine* which in itself engenders still further genres.

Conclusion

> [B]eyond the binary difference that governs the decorum of all codes, beyond the opposition feminine-masculine, beyond bisexuality as well, beyond homosexuality and heterosexuality, which come to the same thing… I would like to believe in the multiplicity of sexually marked voices. I would like to believe in the masses, this indeterminable number of blended voices, this mobile of sexually non-identified sexual marks whose choreography can carry, divide, multiply the body of each 'individual'.[24]

> Tits for me, is an accessory. *(Louella)*

The West's crisis of legitimation is registered in the faltering recognition that genre and gender cannot be accepted complacently; that the law of genre cannot hold. The uncertainties that now disrupt conventional accounts show us that gender, 'like any other identity, is a relational, processual entity'.[25]

To end, however, I want to make it plain that I am not arguing that it is just these *fa'afafines'* marginality that allows for an exceeding, a shattering of the law of masculinity and femininity. Neither is this argument some nostalgic colonial dream of exotic excess. I agree with Butler that what holds for drag queens holds for women and identity in general. That gender itself bears these characteristics as a foundational principle. Rather than being two opposing forces on either side of the binary from one another, masculinity and femininity are integral to each other's identity:

> The breach in the identity and being of the sovereign subject … is a constitutive breaching, a recalling and differentiating within the subject, which calls it into presence … This very breach opens identity to a force field of differences in which the binary divisions … are impossibly implicated.[25]

eight

'As far as sex goes, I don't really think about my body': Young men's corporeal experiences of (hetero)sexual pleasure

LOUISA ALLEN

Academic interest in the male body has flourished over recent years with the publication of numerous articles and edited collections on the topic.[1] This interest has occurred with the emergence of theories of masculinity that have focused the spotlight on men. It has also arisen in response to criticism that a postmodern preoccupation with 'discourse' disregards issues of corporeality and materiality.[2] A popular theme of academic research has been to examine the relationship between sport, gender and male bodies and the way in which sporting ideology and discourses of masculinity construct a notion of ideal masculine physicality.[3] Less frequently, this research has dealt with men's subjective experience of their bodies, in terms of their positive and negative feelings towards them.[4] An issue not addressed by literature on male embodiment is young men's understanding and experience of their bodies in relation to (hetero)sex. The importance of such an investigation lies in understanding how masculine (hetero)sexual subjectivities 'work', and the limitations and advantages they offer for young men's (and young women's) experience of (hetero)sexuality and corporeal pleasure.

In exploring young men's feelings about, and experiences of, their bodies in relation to (hetero)sexual pleasure, data is drawn from a study which examined the (hetero)sexual subjectivities, knowledge and practices of New Zealanders aged seventeen to nineteen years. The 183 young men who participated in the study were volunteers from schools and community training programmes in the Auckland and Hamilton areas. This group was ethnically diverse with around two-thirds still 'at school' and one-third unemployed or in employment training. Data was collected over fourteen months using questionnaires, focus groups, and individual and couple interviews.[5] This multiple-method approach was designed to elicit a diversity of narratives depending upon whether young men were in public (focus group) or private (individual interview) contexts.

In addition to documenting some young men's experiences of corporeal (hetero)sexuality, this chapter aims to conceptualise their experiences in relation to current theory around embodiment and disembodiment. This means determining what corporeal state young men in the research were more likely to experience and how this was experienced by them.

The issue of whether young men are more likely to be sexually embodied or sexually disembodied is a complex one. Within dominant discourses of male heterosexuality, young men's experience of their bodies is said to include guaranteed physical pleasure, facile bodily arousal and perpetual biological readiness for sexual activity. These physical indications, and the fact that young men generally appear to experience few difficulties in achieving sexual pleasure, imply they are 'sexually embodied'.

Simultaneously, masculinity involves a 'detachment' from the body which suggests young men's 'sexual disembodiment'. This can be seen in the literature which describes men's conceptualisation of their bodies as 'machine-like', where the body is treated as an instrument to be used rather than experienced sensually.[6] With reference to the current research findings, I want to explore these competing understandings of corporeal male (hetero)sexuality, and argue they suggest the need for a further concept of 'dys-embodiment'.

In the first section of the chapter I discuss current definitions of the term 'disembodiment' and call for a reformulation of this concept so that Cartesian dualisms are avoided. Drawing on examples of the way in which young men in the research talked about their bodies in relation to (hetero)sex, I argue that what appeared in their talk to be sexual disembodiment, was in fact sexual dys-embodiment. In the second section, I examine young men's experiences of sexual embodiment and the context which made this state possible for some of them. Finally, the way in which the findings point to dys/dis/embodiment as a gendered process and the implications of this for young men's heterosexual subjectivities is discussed.

Reformulating the concept of sexual disembodiment

While issues of embodiment feature prominently in recent literature,[7] there is a paucity of explicit definitions of what this term, and the opposite disembodiment mean. As explanations of young men's experience of disembodiment are especially rare, definitions have been based on research involving young women. The term has generally been used by feminist theorists to denote a woman's detachment from the sensuality of her body.[8] For instance, research proposes that some young women experience minimal physical pleasure during sexual activity because media objectification of female bodies has caused them to be dissatisfied with, and subsequently alienated from, their own.[9] This alienation is expressed in a kind of bodily numbness where pleasurable physical sensation is absent and in an inability to make reference to their bodies in their talk.[11] While there is no research to indicate that young men do not generally find sexual activity corporeally pleasurable, it is possible that they also experience a sensual detachment and/or that their sexual satisfaction is limited by the operation of hegemonic masculinity.

In this kind of definition of disembodiment, the body and the subject (or the 'I' which is socially constructed) are conceived as in Cartesian theory as separate entities. There has been much criticism of this dualistic constitution of subjectivity because of the way it necessarily prioritises mind over body and denies the body agency.[12] Without recognising bodily agency we are confined by a 'logic' that presumes everything is 'mind over matter' and that human dilemmas can be solved by knowledge alone. For instance, Cartesian thought underlies the assumption that when women acknowledge how patriarchal power operates to deny them sexual pleasure, they will be free to experience it. This thinking not only underestimates the power of patriarchal structures, but also the way in which the body is not simply controlled by the mind.

In an attempt to avoid the limitations of Cartesian thought and acknowledge a more complex interweaving of the dualities of mind/body, nature/culture, I have reformulated this general definition of disembodiment in a way that reconceptualises the notion of the body. By 'the body' I do not mean only its flesh, blood, bone or raw materials (its biology), as separate from the socially constructed subject/mind but a necessary interrelation of physiology and culture. In other words, what is knowledge and what is physiology is inseparable in the sense that the body is 'naturally social'.[13] The idea of the subject being 'naturally social' describes the inextricability of biology from the socially constructed subject. With this concept there is no separation between nature/culture, whereby culture works on the raw materials of biology. Biology and culture are undifferentiated, one can not exist without the other to the extent that nature and culture are not a dualism but rather, encompassed by one concept - the 'naturally social'.

Drawing on the work of phenomenologist Merleau-Ponty, it is possible to see the body as a threshold between nature and culture, as the condition and the context through which we are able to have a relation to objects.[14] The body is not an object detached from other objects and subjects, or as Grosz terms it 'a mind somehow cut off from matter and space'.[15] Instead Merleau-Ponty would argue, we are 'subjects being-to-the-world'.[16] It is having and being a body that enables all information and knowledge to be perceived and to have [a] meaning for us.

Utilising this conceptualisation of the body, disembodiment means the loss of sensuality from the body without this involving a splitting of 'I' from physiology. In the case of young men in this research however, loss of sensuality from the body did not involve an inability to experience corporeal sexual pleasure. Sexual disembodiment for these young men involved an absence of acknowledgement of the body and its potential to experience corporeal pleasure beyond what is considered acceptable within the operation of hegemonic masculinity.

SEXUAL DISEMBODIMENT OR DYS-EMBODIMENT?

Identifying if young men in the study were sexually disembodied was a difficult task. This was because their narratives communicated contradictory meanings about whether they did or did not think about their bodies in relation to sexual activity. When asked to think about how their feelings about their bodies might influence their sexual activity, young men in the focus groups and individual interviews denied being consciously aware of their bodies. The response typically provided was 'I don't really think about it', or they immediately took up the subject position of their girlfriend offering her thoughts about their body. In this way, these young men distanced themselves from subjective feelings and thoughts about their bodies implying they were *disembodied*. Three-quarters of the young men who participated in the individual interviews provided this *seemingly* disembodied response by claiming they were not concerned with their bodies:

Ashby Uhm, I don't know. As far as sex goes, I don't really think about my body. (II, AS,17)[17]

Tim How I feel about my body? … no I feel … she's fine with my body and that's all that really matters. I'm like not having sex with myself so I don't really care how I look (*laugh*), so I mean if she is happy with my body then there is no problem. (II, NAS, 18)

Neil No, no, I don't feel, I just don't feel anything about it, sort of over cocky you know 'Oh I've got a good body' so I just don't care. My body's just there and it doesn't worry me you know. (II, NAS, 17)

Chris I don't think that it matters. I mean I don't really care what my body looks like. I do care what Cam thinks my body looks like (*stabs the table with his finger for emphasis*). Like so I always ask Cam, I, I, I oh not always but I do on occasion ask Cam, you know, 'Am I good enough for you?' (II, NAS, 19)

This sense of not really caring about their bodies was also communicated in the questionnaire. Answers to the question 'what do you do most and least with your body'? indicated young men generally took a neutral stance on their bodies. In other words, they were highly unlikely to say that they always thought their body was 'nice' or that they always 'criticised it'. This absence of a tendency towards a positive or negative perception appears to support the notion that young men were concerned with their bodies.

However, despite alleging when asked directly, that they 'don't think' and 'don't care' about their bodies, the six young men who participated in the interviews revealed that they did in fact think about them and these thoughts centred around anxieties about their bodies. In these instances young men spoke of their body's inadequacies, making a mental comparison with dominant conceptions of the 'perfect' male body. Their references to 'small biceps', 'lack of muscle' or not being 'toned' and being 'short', all indicated a comparison of themselves with a socially constituted 'ideal' model generally 'characterised by a well developed chest, rippling arm muscles and a 'washboard stomach'.[18] The following extracts come from individual and couple interviews with men who were currently in a relationship.

Tim explained that before he met his girlfriend: 'I thought my body was ugly'. (II, NAS, 18)

Giving an appraisal of his body Peter said: 'Well, my biceps aren't that big and (*laugh*) and you know I'm not well toned'. (II, NAS, 18)

Chris (II, NAS, 19), referring to his girlfriend seeing his body, described how his insecurities about his body meant that 'some days I just don't, I just don't want her to see me'. A little further into the interview Chris explained explicitly that this was because:

> Just uhm a feeling of inadequacy because like, you know like I feel that, I feel that Cam [his girlfriend] is so amazing that I'm not really good enough, like that's just like a I dunno it's probably irrational but you know it's like you really, really, really want to make the other person happy and like if you don't have say Carlos Spencer's body (*laugh*) … Cam has a huge crush on Carlos Spencer.

Indicating some feelings of insecurity about how attractive his girlfriend found his body, Neil (CA, NAS, 17) described how he thought she wanted him to be more stereotypically masculine:

> I mean sure there's different things that you want on everyone. I mean I am sure Nina wishes that I was a bit more muscular or what ever else …

After saying he didn't care about his body, Ashby revealed his concern about being 'too short', and the feeling that he had to compensate for this with extra muscle in order to 'look good' and be a good sportsman.

> *Interviewer* So going to the gym and doing weights and stuff like that is to make you feel better or … why do you do it?
>
> *Ashby* Really it's for sports but uhm it does have, it does make you look better and stuff like that. But uhm my basic uhm motivation uhm is just for sport cos I'm a bit on the short side so I've got to, you know, I've got to try and make myself bigger. (II, AS, 17)

The fact that some of the young men in the study thought about or worried about their bodies, even though when questioned directly they maintained that they did not, might be explained by the operation of hegemonic masculinity. Hegemonic masculinity involves young men denying or protecting their own 'vulnerability', where vulnerability entails [their] failure to achieve dominant perceptions of masculinity.[19] For young men in this study, admitting that their bodies were 'inadequate' meant exposing their vulnerability. This is because within the operation of hegemonic masculinity successful men are constituted as 'invincible', and have strong imposing bodies that match this image. Referring to their bodies, except in relation to sport, or drawing attention to their worries about them, threatened to sabotage their achievement of an appropriately masculine identity.

When disembodiment has been documented in research on young women, an absence of 'the body' in their talk has been noted.[20] However, the young men in this study acknowledged their bodies, albeit in negative ways, indicating their awareness of their corporeality. There was also no evidence of their lack of corporeal sexual pleasure, which has typically been associated with the disembodiment of young women. Speaking of sexual pleasure as an experience that was easy and 'guaranteed' for them, Tim and Chris, made comments which were typical of other young men in the research:

Tim … if I wanted to ejaculate I could probably just do so in less than a minute. (II, NAS, 18)

Chris … a guy is sort of almost guaranteed to feel good [having sex] you know, feel the same in the end anyway so. (II, NAS, 19)

The corporeal awareness and reference to physical sexual pleasure in young men's talk indicated that they were not sexually disembodied. A better way of conceptualising these young men's experiences of their bodies might be to use the term sexual dys-embodiment. Williams utilises the term dys-embodiment to describe 'embodiment in a dysfunctional state'.[21] He takes 'dys' from the Greek prefix signifying 'bad', 'hard', or 'ill' as it is present in words such as 'dysfunctional', and applies it to the bodily state chronically ill patients often encounter: '… the painful body emerges as 'thing like'; 'it 'betrays' us and we may feel alienated and estranged from it as a consequence'.[22]

While young men's awareness of their bodies might be seen to indicate their embodiment, their relationship with them was characterised by dys-embodiment. The dissatisfaction with their bodies revealed by the young men above indicated a negative relationship distorted by dominant perceptions of masculine bodily 'perfection'. Awareness of their bodies did not equate with positive embodiment, but led to feelings of insecurity and anxiety about not being physically 'good enough'.

Similarly, their talk about physical sexual pleasure described an experience that was constrained by dominant discourses of male heterosexuality. Tim's claim that he could 'ejaculate' if he wanted to 'in less than a minute' communicated a sensual detachment from this experience, as if this were a physical achievement rather than a truly pleasurable activity. Chris's statement that 'a guy is almost always guaranteed to feel good in the end anyway' also implied a mechanical rather than sensual quality to corporeal sexual pleasure. These narratives might be described as dys-embodied in that such corporeal sexual pleasure is limited by dominant discourses that constitute only certain ways of experiencing bodily pleasure as appropriate. In these young men's talk, the body is conceptualised as a mechanical instrument which will inevitably provide them with sexual pleasure rather than a pool of potential pleasure which might be explored. Subsequently, certain sexual acts (homosexual, female penetration of the male) are off limits because they are not sanctioned within the operation of hegemonic masculinity as appropriately masculine.

Young men's narratives of sexual embodiment

While at times the young men in this study indicated they were dys-embodied in their experience of sexual pleasure, at others their talk indicated sexual embodiment. Some authors have used 'embodied' simply to refer to possessing a 'bodily' form. This is apparent in Williams's discussion of illness and the relationship this forces subjects to have with their body. He describes the relationship as '… a shift from an initial state of embodiment, one in which the body is largely taken-for-granted in the course of everyday life' to a recognition of the way in which the ill person's body has let them down.[23] While to be 'embodied' within this definition does not require the subject's conscious acknowledgement of their body, for other theorists, this process of recognition is integral to their use of the term. For example, Holland *et al.*[24] talk about the importance for young women of recognising the differencc between what Rich[25] has described as 'the body' and 'my body'. It is only by recognising this difference that young women are able to experience an embodied sexuality. Holland *et al.* argue that it is a lack of critical consciousness in distinguishing between dominant conceptions of 'appropriate' feminine bodies and their own corporeality that leaves young women living a 'disembodied' femininity.[26]

Arguably, an empowering embodiment for young men also requires their acknowledgement of the discursive construction of their bodies. Dominant discourses supporting hegemonic masculinity construct the male body as an 'unfeeling machine' which men use to demonstrate power and subsequently attain successful masculine identity.[27] Being embodied for young men, therefore, could require them to transgress dominant discourses of masculinity by acknowledging their own bodies and the range of their unrealised sensual potential in unconventional ways. In this chapter, I use 'embodied' to mean *recognition* of the presence and sensuality of the body in ways that deviate from dominant discourses of masculinity.

Being embodied for young men in the study was about escaping dominant discourses of male sexuality in which sexual activity was experienced corporeally as 'self-gratifying' or as a 'release'. As indicated by Tim and Chris above, in dominant discourses young men's bodies are represented as machines that simply 'do sex' in order to achieve orgasm, but are not experienced sensually by them. Sensuality for some young men in the research was accessed through emotional feelings which heightened bodily satisfaction in sexual activity. In the following extracts, young men illustrate this connection between emotional and bodily satisfaction. Chris, George and Ashby (all involved in heterosexual relationships) described in the individual interviews how casual sex was different from sex in more enduring relationships.

Here, Chris talked about his first sexual experience with his girlfriend, Cam, as better than other casual sexual experiences he'd had, because of the emotion he felt for her.

Interviewer So what was sex like the first time with Cam?
Chris … it went well, it was like astounding, wow it was good you know uhm (*laugh*).
Interviewer Better than previous times?
Chris Yes.
Interviewer So better than one-night stands?
Chris It was better, it was just like it made sex worthwhile, like sex for me it wasn't worthwhile before, it doesn't give you anything like you, it didn't make you, it didn't make you feel particularly good or anything and like sex with Cam is really good.
Interviewer So what's different?
Chris I'm sure there must have been much more emotion in there, like there was real caring … like there wasn't … like this isn't because of sex, this was because, just because I feel good with her *(stabs finger into table for definition)* … Yeah sex for sex sake isn't worthwhile. (II, NAS, 19)

Speaking about why sex with his girlfriend, Ngaire, was 'fun' and 'better' than a one night stand, George explained:

> You know that you really know them, like before [with one night stands] it was like turned on but you never get to know them or who they were or how they felt about such and such a thing … it's best if you can get to know them that's the fun … the sex is better yeah. (II, NAS, 19)

Ashby described how sexual intercourse with his long-term girlfriend, Becky, was more 'intimate' and 'comfortable' because of his feelings for her, where as in a 'one-night stand' for him sex was simply about lust:

> Uhm it's more intimate generally [in a long term relationship] uhm … yeah … yeah, yeah cause like I care about her and stuff like that … I'm just more comfortable with Becky (*small laugh*). It's like uhm with the others it's just more lust yeah. (II, AS, 17)

The link between emotions and a heightened corporeal sensation is apparent in each of these interviews. For Chris, the presence of 'much more emotion' in his relationship with his girlfriend made sex as he described it 'astounding'. Similarly for Ashby, caring about Becky made his sexual experiences more 'intimate' and 'comfortable' than with 'a one-night stand'. Sex was 'better' for George because 'getting to know someone' is what produces 'the fun'. The embodiment these young men displayed was enabled by taking up alternative subject positions in those discourses which construct male bodies as separated from emotion and machine-like in their procurement of gratification. Instead, embodiment for these young men came from the way an acknowledgement of their emotions enabled them to draw greater pleasure from their bodies. In a sense, their emotions were a source of increased physical pleasure for them.

Embodied narratives were also revealed in answers to a survey question which asked subjects to complete the sentence 'what I find pleasurable about sexual activity is …'. Young men's embodiment was revealed in their reports of pleasurable corporeal feelings that were inextricably bound with emotional 'intimacy', 'closeness' and 'the thought of being with someone you love'. Below are some descriptions of what these young men found pleasurable about sexual activity:

> The intimacy and the stimulation. (Q, NAS, 19)
> Talking and being touched by my partner. (Q, AS, 17)
> Close feeling, orgasm. (Q, AS, 17)
> The presence (physical and mental) of a female. Being physically stimulated. (Q, AS, 18)
> The intimacy and the pleasure. (Q, AS, 17)
> Making love to the person that you love. Not just getting satisfied physically but the whole being. (Q, NAS, 18)
> Intercourse and oral sex. The thought of being with someone you love. (Q, AS, 18)

Here the links between emotion ('the intimacy', 'love') and physical pleasure ('orgasm', 'getting satisfied physically') are made. Because the study preserved the interviewees' anonymity, I could not explore this relationship further. However, the answers suggest these young men appeared to experience embodiment. For young men in this research, embodiment was about treating the body as connected with emotions not constituted as 'appropriately masculine' and allowing those emotions to intensify pleasurable corporeal sensation.

What enabled these young men to speak in embodied ways while other young men did not seems to be that the former shared a common experience. Each had been in a long-term relationship in which they professed having some emotional investment. Both George and Chris, for example, proclaimed that they 'loved' their girlfriends while Ashby explained, 'I just like being around her, and she's really good to me and that's what I like about it [the relationship]'.

Entering into relationships often forces a recognition of young men's feelings since, as Holland *et al.* argue, 'negotiating sexual encounters can engage their emotions, connect them to their need for affection, and render visible their dependence on women'.[28] Being in a relationship provided some young men with a context in which they could legitimately connect their feelings, enabling them to experience the connection between their bodies and such feelings.

EMBODIMENT AND DYS-EMBODIMENT AS GENDERED PROCESSES

For young men, the states of sexual embodiment and dys-embodiment can be seen to be gendered because they are inextricably tied to the operation of hegemonic masculinity. In this study young men's sexual dys-embodiment was seen in the way they recounted experiences of sexual pleasure. These descriptions produced bodies that were emotionally detached and automated. Such representations attest to hegemonic masculinity's power in encouraging young men to produce themselves in ways that are 'appropriately' masculine.

Young men's sexual embodiment was also a gendered state achieved through gendered processes. Sexual embodiment for young men in this research involved exploring a bodily sensuality beyond the boundaries of hegemonic masculinity. This sensuality was accessed by an emotional attachment to their sexual partner which subsequently increased pleasurable bodily sensations for them. In acknowledging and enjoying their emotional investment in sexual activity, young men took up alternative subject positions within dominant discourses of male heterosexuality.

The implications of sexual embodiment for young men are varied and perhaps far reaching. On the one hand, being sexually embodied opens a whole realm of potentially new ways of expressing (hetero)sexual masculinity and experiencing corporeal sexual pleasure. Young men who experience sexual embodiment are likely to be less restricted by the sexual acts and expressions which might bring them physical pleasure. The flip side of this 'freedom' however is that it potentially connects young men with vulnerability in the face of hegemonic masculinity's operation. Speaking and focusing on their bodies in ways that transgress dominant discourses of masculinity risk young men's achievement of attaining 'appropriate' masculinity. At the same time, being sexually embodied suggests creating space within the discourses of dominant masculinity which (re)produce male power and have negative consequences for young women. It might be ventured then, that young men's sexual embodiment could offer new ways of experiencing (hetero) sexual relationships that have positive consequences (sexual or otherwise) for both genders.

nine

Young Pakeha Men's Conceptions of Health, Illness and Health Care

ANTHONY M. O'CONNOR

This chapter explores the relationship between gender and health in the context of the lives of some Pakeha men aged fifteen to twenty-four years ('Pakeha' meaning a person of predominantly European descent').[1] The work presented here is based on a study that examined other works in the social sciences of health, as well as primary qualitative and quantitative data collected by questionnaire, interview and newspaper analysis. Some standard census questions and the SF-36 self-rating of health survey were included in the questionnaire to provide an indication as to the health and socio-economic status of the respondents. The outcome of this work shows how conceptions and practices of masculinity in New Zealand affect the way young men think about and care for their health, and how their health and health-related practices in turn affect their masculinity.[2]

Background

The contemporary Western health sciences favour a holistic 'bio-psycho-social' view of health that identifies biological, psychological and social forces as having a determinant role in the health of the individual and population group.[3] This view of health recognises that biological and social forces interact with and have effect on each other. Developmental processes and socialisation help individuals develop an understanding of the body, health and illness. The sociocultural context gives meaning to biological phenomena, and it also contributes to the environment in which biological phenomena have the potential to be expressed. The relationship is not one-way, however, as biology provides the potential for sociocultural interaction – for example, the physiological capacity for communication and cognition affords the capacity for social interaction. In the context of health and illness then, social structures are at the confluence of biological forces.[4] In recognising the interplay of biology and society in health, one must remain aware that there are multiple concepts of 'health' that carry through to influence conceptions of what 'healthy' behaviours may be.[5]

Like other forms of practice, health-related behaviours are influenced by an individual's health status, social structures and agency.[6] Health research is coming to recognise the importance of choice and compulsion in health behaviour because health belief models are increasingly being shown as poor predictors of health-related behaviours.[7] For example, Cameron and Bernardes found amongst a group of men suffering from prostatitis, a need to respond to their suffering differentially, depending on the 'role' they were trying to fulfil (for example as husband, friend or employee) as well as in response to the social setting.[8] Thus, the process of behavioural response revealed the compulsion and choices that underlie the role gender plays in health-related behaviour.

Like Cameron and Bernardes,[9] Connell argues that rather than establish practice *types*, we need to focus on the *process* and relationships in which men (and women) conduct gendered lives. For him, gender should be viewed as a 'configuration of practice' simultaneously positioned in a number of structures and relationships based around power, production relations, and emotional attachment.[10] Connell also argues that a hegemonic form of masculinity embodies the currently accepted answer to the congruence between dominant forms of masculinity and the associated domination of the social hierarchy. Individual men's masculinity can be undermined and challenged at any time because the social world is fluid, which renders identity and relationships of power vulnerable to change. Therefore, dominance plays a very large part in the structuring of masculine gendered practices and identity.

Not only gender, but also ethnicity and age are recognised as important predictors of health status.[11] However, gender, ethnicity and age should not be considered as creating generic bodies of health-related behaviours and types. Rather, gender, ethnicity and age should be thought of as being among a variety of factors 'that together produce the plurality of patterns of dispositions, constraints and choices that are identifiable in complex modern settings'.[12]

James and Saville-Smith quote Connell's identification of the struggle for young working-class men to display authority and control in an (Australian) adult and bourgeois-dominated world:

> The points on which the issue of control is fought out, smoking, drinking, driving, fucking, foul language and physical aggression, are an inextricable mixture of claims to adulthood and claims to masculinity. Their barrenness reflects the very limited claims that can be made by people who, because of the age and class structure, have very few resources.[13]

As is further discussed below, for young men, especially those with limited financial capital and cultural claims to masculinity, demonstrating control over one's own body is an immediately accessible medium for the demonstration of masculinity. The demonstration of masculinity through practices such as drinking and displays of physical strength and domination carries potentially negative health consequences; such practices may encourage denial of pain

Rank	Men	Women
1	Injury (unintentional)	Cancer
2	Cancer	Infant conditions
3	Injury (intentional)	Other chronic diseases
4	Cardio-vascular disease	Injury (unintentional)
5	Infant conditions	Injury (intentional)

Table 1. Comparison of contemporary leading causes of presenescent (under 65 years of age) mortality of men and women in New Zealand (adapted from Ministry of Health 1999:141).

and suffering and delay a request for help when it is needed. This may underlie young men's particularly poor injury record (Table 1). Indeed, the greatest gap between male and female mortality rates in New Zealand is in the fifteen to twenty-four year age bracket due to greater unintentional and intentional injury of men.[14] In the North Health region, three times more men than women die from, or present for health care with injuries sustained through violence, motor vehicle accidents and suicide.

The respondents to this study report a wide variety of practices and personal experiences in relation to health, illness and health care. Nevertheless, themes running through the respondents' conceptions and reported behaviours can be identified. The results that reveal these themes will be presented next, followed by a discussion and some conclusions.

Results

The Sample Group

Sixty respondents to this study were aged between fifteen and twenty-four years with a mean age of twenty-one years. All were urban men in paid employment who had completed seventh form or had some tertiary education. While some remained financially dependent, others earned above the average full-time wage. Eighty-eight per cent of the respondents' households had an annual income above $30,000, that figure being just below the average full-time wage in New Zealand. By comparison, the Northern Region as a whole, from where the sample was drawn, has only 49 per cent of households with an income above $30,000 per annum.[15] Seventeen respondents were in a committed relationship and two were married. None had dependents, although four were preparing for the support of dependents. Seven noted their sexual orientation as bisexual. Table 2 shows significant biographic, accommodation and health details of the young men who took part in this study.

A comparison of the respondents' self-rated health to a nationally

Table 2: Biographic details of the respondents referred to in the text

Respondent	Age	Relationship Status	Resides in	Perceived Global Health Status	Perceived Health Care Effort Made
Mr 2	24	single	family member's house	good	fair
Mr 3	24	committed relationship	rental accommodation	good	fair
Mr 5	23	single	family member's house	good	fair
Mr 8	21	single a	family member's house	very good	fair
Mr 10	22	single	own home	good (had crossed out 'excellent')	fair
Mr 11	22	committed relationship	family member's house	excellent	excellent
Mr 14	23	committed relationship	family member's house	good	good
Mr 15	24	committed relationship	rental accommodation	very good	very good
Mr 19	23	single	family member's house	excellent	very good
Mr 22	20	committed relationship	family member's house	very good	poor
Mr 24	24	single	rental accommodation	good	fair
Mr 26	22	committed relationship	family member's house	good	fair
Mr 30	22	single	family member's house	very good	fair
Mr 31	20	single	family member's house	fair	fair
Mr 35	20	single	rental accommodation	fair	poor
Mr 38	17	single	family member's house	good	poor
Mr 40	17	single	family member's house	excellent	very good
Mr 44	19	committed relationship	rental accommodation	fair	good
Mr 45	19	single	rental accommodation	good	fair
Mr 46	19	single	family member's house	fair	poor
Mr 47	18	single	family member's house	very good	fair
Mr 53	19	single	family member's house	very good	excellent
Mr 55	17	committed relationship	family member's house	good	fair
Mr 56	19	single	family member's house	excellent	very good
Mr 57	19	single	family member's house	good	good
Mr 59	18	single	rental accommodation	fair	good
Mr 60	24	committed relationship	rental accommodation	fair	fair

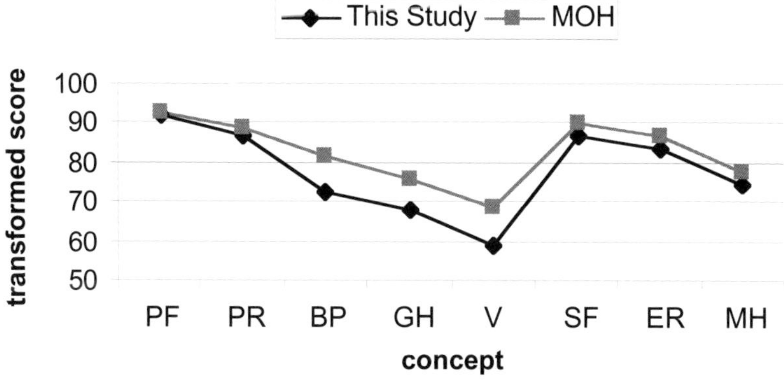

Figure 1. Comparison of nationally representative mean SF-36 scores of men of all ethnicities in the 15–24 years age group (Ministry of Health 1999) and mean scores obtained from this study's sample group. PF, physical functioning; PR physical role; BP bodily pain; GH general health; V vitality; SF social functioning; ER emotional role; MH mental health.

representative sample of men aged fifteen to twenty-four of all ethnicities is shown by Figure 1.[16] This shows that the men rate their health poorly in general, and poorer than what is expected of a sample of men with indicators of an average to above-average socio-economic status.[17] A comparison between the sample group and a sample of haemophilia sufferers (n = 193, of whom 184 were men) again shows that the sample group rate their health poorly (Figure 2). The haemophilia sufferers were mainly young, married Pakeha males living in a family situation who earned a wage that met their living expenses.[18]

Conceptions of 'Health'

The respondents were asked: 'What does the word "health" mean to you?' A theme running through the men's conceptions of health is that every respondent recognised the physical dimension of health as important. Mr 19, for example, saw health as 'physical fitness', while 72 per cent of respondents elaborated on this with multifaceted responses such as 'physical and mental well-being' (Mr 22).

While most of the respondents viewed health as a holistic concept, their concepts of health and health care were greatly influenced by the demonstration of great fitness, and strength of sportsmen. Among sports rugby is central to the respondents' conceptions of health and masculinity; those who identified an exemplar of men's health only ever identified the All Blacks in particular, and élite sportsmen in general. But not only were sportsmen a standard against which the respondents measured their health, they also learnt about health from sportsmen. Mr 60 said, 'You can just see it in the players you know. You can see the fitness level they are at, compared to where the body can go …'. The respondents' identification of rugby players as embodying the ideal of men's health furthers the recognition of rugby's symbolic dominance within discourses of masculinity. Phillips reviews the gendered, social and political history of Pakeha men in New Zealand which, he argues, is inextricably connected with the cultivated emergence of rugby as the national game.[19]

All Black Todd Blackadder is one such athlete who influences the young men's knowledge and conceptions of health. He was the subject of a newspaper special feature which went to press soon after he was chosen as All Black captain.[20] It noted that a great attraction for promoting Blackadder to the All Black captaincy was his back-to-basics approach. The feature reads:

> Team-mate Matt Sexton says, 'Blackadder has the characteristics of a great Canterbury player. He's got that real sort of hard background, and that's the way he plays, he loves the hard graft' … Commentators and arm chair fans like his uncomplicated style. He reportedly summed up his footballing approach after watching a sports psychology video with the national sevens team … 'It's all bullshit, mate. You just run, tackle, and run and tackle some more.'[21]

Blackadder's beliefs that psychology and anything other than muscle power are vacuous, and the romanticism of his qualities as a good bloke, are detrimental to health promotion. Characteristics of 'the good bloke' suppress awareness of pain and the recognition of the mind and body as vulnerable; this may lead to the exacerbation and increased frequency of certain types of injury and illness among men.

Popular culture and the media do not portray the fact that sports are the reason for many health problems. Messner notes the irony in that even though professional sportsmen in the United States embody the ideal of masculine strength and health, they have an average life expectancy of fifty-six years, fifteen years less than the average for other men in the United States.[22] Park points to the fact that, in the mid 1990s, half of the accident compensation payments in New Zealand were claimed by players in five fields of sport, of which half were rugby players.[23] One respondent to this study, Mr 5, 'gave up playing rugby' with the intention of improving his health.

The responses of some men in this study are attributable to what each as an individual wants to do or does in this day-to-day life: 'Feeling comfortable with yourself, being able to do what you want,' said Mr 10 on the theme of physical health. Viewing health as providing the capacity to do what one wants is associated with placing more importance on some aspects of it than others. Three men referred to spirituality as being important. Two of them made reference to being Christians and the other practises yoga. For Mr 46, who is an actor, having a toned body and a clear voice are most important.

Concepts of health change in response to intimacy, life experience and life course. Mr 15 explained to me how he became aware of mental health: 'Yeah,

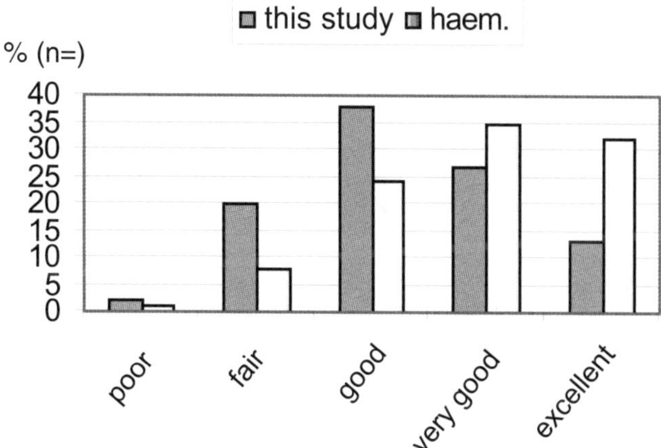

Figure 2. Comparison between the global health status of respondents to this study and a group of haemophilia sufferers. (Park 2000)

basically what brought me to an awareness of mental health is having psychotic girlfriends. I went along to a couple of counselling sessions just to support them, and they affected me so much I had to go to counselling myself.' Several respondents noted their personal hygiene improved when they entered intimate relationships, and one respondent (Mr 37) noted that he made an effort to lose weight to improve 'bedroom aesthetics'.

The more eloquent definitions of health provided by some respondents sometimes reflected their education level. Mr 15, for example, discussed health from a Maori perspective, Hauora,[24] which he became familiar with as part of his student-teacher education. During his interview, Mr 15 demonstrated how health education has beneficial results. His education has enabled him to reflect upon, make sense of, and articulate his views on health and illness. This skill is essential in order to ask for health care and advice from friends, family, and health professionals. However, there was not a significant statistical relationship between education level and perceived health status in the sample.

While formal education has great benefits and is shown to be effective in allowing people to express conceptions of health and illness, ten of the eleven respondents interviewed noted that their formal health education had been minimal or not remembered at all. Peers, family, the media and personal experience are at least as important sources of information about health, illness and health care as formal education. For fifty-nine of the sixty respondents, their own lived experiences were the most important influences in their learning about health and illness, followed by their peers' experiences and images in the media. Health, illness and health care is something they just 'felt' and 'did' rather than thought about. For example, Mr 57 defined sickness as 'not 100 per cent normal, and Mr 47, 'unwell?!!, sick!?'. For the most part, information about health, illness and health-care within the sample were absorbed unconsciously and reflected in day-to-day thought and behaviour:

Interviewer How do you remember learning about health and illness as a kid?
Mr 46 I don't, I don't remember how, it just comes about I guess, um … I don't remember anything from primary school, nothing from my parents. I actually have no idea how you come to learn about health or illness.

Conceptions of 'Sickness'

Many of the themes running through the respondents' concepts of sickness were similar to those raised in discussions about 'health'. Again, physical effects dominate the definitions of sickness. Twenty-nine respondents explicitly referred to the physical, for example, Mr 2 had 'a sense of feeling physically unwell'. Eleven respondents explicitly referred to emotions and/or psychology, Mr 31 defining sickness as 'physically or mentally ill, vomit'. Half of the respondents referred to sickness as the opposite of health.

Most respondents also defined sickness as disrupting what they wanted to do, or be. Sickness was kept as private as possible, with respondents preferring not to affect or engage others in their experience of sickness. Mr 40, for example, defined sickness as 'being incapacitated and unable to perform your normal duties'. Sickness and injury interrupted the ability to lead lives they would have chosen if they had had good health.

There probably is an important difference in the men's conceptions of 'illness' as opposed to 'injury'.[25] The difference between injury and sickness was not queried, as I was not aware of this important distinction during the questionnaire and interview data collection phase of the research. However, there are some indications as to how the respondents think of injury in the data. When a respondent spoke of illness during the focus group, the other men listened without comment until he had finished speaking. However, when a participant spoke of injury, the conversation was animated with jokes, jibes and laughter. For example:

Interviewer I haven't asked you about hospitals actually. What's your experience of hospitals?
Mr 60 Yeah, I've been in there heaps: broken collarbone, broken hand, concussion, broken nose, broken thumb … (*the group responded to this with laughter*).
Interviewer Is that right, you've had all that happen to you?
Mr 60 I've had shit loads (*group laughter*) … I just live life on the edge.
Interviewer Doing what?
Mr 60 If someone said to me 'I bet you can't jump over that', Oh fuck off! (*laughs*), ahhh!!! (*makes jumping action*). You know, you only live once. I broke my collarbone when I was running playing paintball

> and I missed the bridge and *whack* (*laughs*). Yeah, I just live life on the edge.

There were two pieces of anecdotal evidence in the primary data that revealed non-physical dimensions to the experience of illness and injury particularly explicitly. They are as follows.

Mr 53's understanding of existential issues was disrupted by a car accident. This car accident led Mr 53 to a realisation of his own mortality and to find security in a 'Supernatural Being' more permanent than his own body. The way in which he thought about existential issues before the accident did not provide him with satisfactory ways in which to respond to issues brought up by the car crash. After the accident his thoughts turned to 'what life *really* is about and seek[ing] God *more*', which provided him with solace.

Mr 35's traumatic experience has had negative health consequences. It has also led him to reassess his identity. He feels as though he needs drugs to help him cope with his experience. He said: 'Losing a girlfriend led me to have a loss of where I felt I belonged in the world. Depression resulting in an increase in the use of substances that I know are hurting my body'. Mr 35's identity was disrupted by an event which he felt could not, or should not, happen to him as he understood himself to be. He is effecting control over his bodily sensations to try and control psychological and emotional trauma over which he feels he has no control: 'Depression causing me to want to feel a little physical pain, perhaps to dull emotional pain'.

Conceptions of Health Care

The respondents' answers to the question 'Compared to other men of my age group the effort I make to look after my health is: poor, fair, good, very good, excellent' were divided into two groups with close to half the respondents in each in order to aid intra-sample analyses. Figure 3 compares how the respondents in the low effort group (n=34) and high effort group (n=26) perceived their global health status. The correspondence between perceived health status and effort made is statistically significant (chi square 9.94, d.f.=1, $p<0.05$). Thus, there is a perception of self-responsibility for health status and care among the respondents, but this self-responsibility is not absolute, as will be discussed below. Comparing Figures 2 and 3 shows that the 'high effort' group and the haemophilia sufferers rate their health similarly. This 'high effort' group of respondents shows similar ratings of health to the Ministry of Health sample of males aged fifteen to twenty-four of all ethnicities (Figure 4).[26]

Day-to-day health care practices focused on physical health, as did the recourse measures when the men felt 'slightly' or 'really' sick. Eating healthy food and getting exercise were the most common ways in which the respondents practise health care. When they feel slightly sick, getting exercise or resting is commonly practised. Many of the respondents took 'tonics' such as a cup of

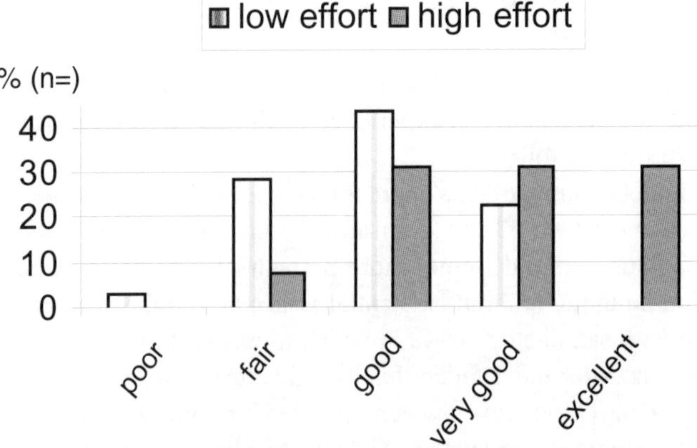

Figure 3. Comparison of global health status between those who see the *effort* they make to practise health care to be good, very good, or excellent, to those who see their health care as poor or fair. The question was worded 'Compared to other men of my age group, the effort I make to look after my health is: …'

tea, garlic, echinacea, or oranges. These remedies were just as popular as over-the-counter medicines. When they felt really sick, health care practices included 'stay in bed and sleep' (Mr 8); 'Eat well – veggies steamed with garlic, runny noses I use tissues – *no sniffing* – and a small bowl [a smoker's pipe stoked with cannabis] to smoke' (Mr 15); and 'Sleep, keep warm, talk to friends and see what they suggest' (Mr 45). Also, when they felt really sick, 92 per cent of the respondents did something about it, but only 55 per cent said they sought medical advice. In the last twelve months, 67 per cent of the respondents had visited a general practitioner. This is a little less than Parr *et al.*'s finding that 75 per cent of men and women aged between fifteen and twenty-four had visited a general practitioner in the previous twelve months.[27] In both studies, general practitioners were the most visited health professional.

Many respondents predicted that their health care would improve when they become involved in an intimate relationship. Mr 3 would improve his health 'if I was seriously contending someone because I would be trying to make myself look more viable …'. During the focus group there was general discussion about how their health care would improve if they became husbands or fathers. There was consensus that they would have to be healthy to provide for the family. They also agreed that there would be extra reason to be healthy if there was somebody else to be healthy for. They felt as though they already had the necessary knowledge about health and health care, but there was no need for this knowledge to be implemented in their lives now.

The respondents referred to men not having a great interest in health care practices. Such practices symbolised a difference between men and women. As Mr 3 put it: 'Guys don't want to look feminine.' Mr 24 said, '…women

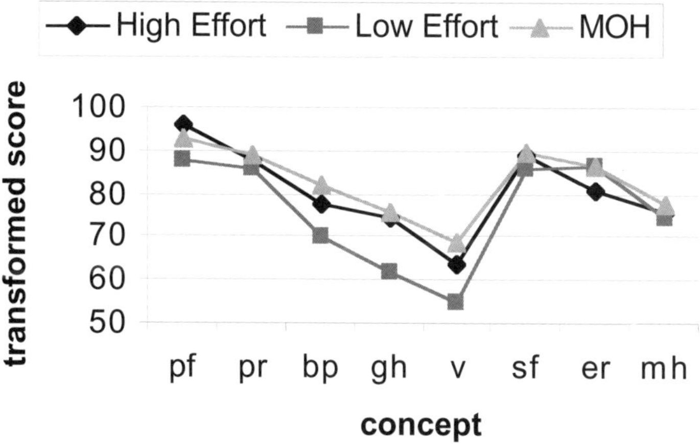

Figure 4. Comparison of mean SF-36 scores between Ministry of Health (1999) and the respondents to this study who rate their health keeping as very good or excellent, and those respondents who rate their health keeping as good, fair or poor.

want to take more care than men, mainly because I think it is the subculture in New Zealand, being a man sort of thing. I can put up with a bit of pain or what have you, looking tough, she'll be right mate, definitely'. Stoicism underlies many of the respondents' hesitance towards practising health care. Seven respondents make an effort to ignore symptoms when they feel either 'slightly' or 'really' sick. Mr 11, for example, said he would 'Tell myself to get over it and try to forget it.'

The men lose autonomy and authority over their actions and themselves when nursing sickness and injury, especially when seeking health care from experts. Mr 26 said he was reluctant to seek medical care when sick,

> because your body is the one thing in life that you can have control over and when you go to the doctor's you have to let them do what they want to your body. You don't know what they are doing, you lose control over your own body.

Socio-economic concerns also discouraged the respondents from taking health care, particularly when doing so involved a disruption to their performance as employee, team-mate, or student. Health care might require spending money that they would not spend otherwise, and not performing as well as they like at their place of work, sport, or study. Fulfilling a felt obligation to sports teams and employers, and facing competition in the workplace and educational institutions are frequently mentioned as reasons to not want to take the time to practise health care.

Medical professionals may be the main source of health care and advice, but they are not the only source. Both personal and secondhand experience contribute to men's knowledge about health, illness and health care practices.

Behaviour	Low Health Status n=36	High Health Status n=24	Chi Square Significance
Will have sex without a condom with a partner of unknown STI status	(%) 20	(%) 0	(d.f.=1) p<0.05
Reside in family member's house	58	88	P<0.05
Current tobacco smoker	36	0	P<0.05
Current user of illegal drugs	56	21	P<0.05

Table 3. The statistically significant relationships between health-related behaviours and perceived health status.

Mr 31 told how his cannabis smoking 'changed because I was beginning to lack motivation etc. and my brain wasn't functioning as it should so I cut down quite a bit'. Mr 24's health care practice has been affected by his desire to lose weight, and a health scare that his boss had:

> Lately I have started trying to not drink as much beer. If I am going to go out and drink I will generally get a couple of bottles of wine or something, mainly because apparently beer is more fattening than wine (*laughs*). My boss had a bit of a scare not long ago and the doctor urged him to drink wine instead of beer, so I have kind of taken that on board a bit.

Maintaining good mental health was not given as a reason for practising health care, even though it is fairly widely accepted that health care practices said to benefit physical health may also benefit mental health. Despite twenty-three respondents reporting factors such as lack of sleep, stress, mental sickness and depression being causes of sickness, mental health care was not a concern. Some reported they used illegal drugs or alcohol when they were stressed mentally or emotionally. Only one respondent took measures to reduce mental and emotional stress other than illegal drugs or alcohol. Mr 15, a computer network manager, expressed the opinion of several others in saying, 'We [referring to Pakeha men in general] are very competitive and that can make things quite stressful, like at work'.

The men's lack of awareness of mental health is of particular concern given New Zealand's high suicide rate and that many of the respondents noted mental stress as a cause of sickness. One respondent explicitly referred to using drugs and alcohol to control what he perceived to be quite severe emotional and psychological pain. Raeburn and Sidaway argue that an inability to express a need for help, and an inability to cope are effects of stoicism and 'toughing it out' for which men are traditionally respected in New Zealand.[28]

The gendering of health-related practices leads to a deterioration of perceived health status when young men move away from the family home. Table 3 shows that there is a significant relationship between living

Behaviour	Low Effort n=33 (%)	High Effort n= 26 (%)	Chi Square Significance (d.f.=1)
Will have sex without a condom with a partner of unknown STI status	15	0	P<0.05
Reside in family member's house	65	77	n.s.
Current tobacco smoker	29	12	n.s
Current user of illegal drugs	44	39	n.s.

Table 4. The percentage of respondents who perform the indicated health-related behaviours grouped by their perceived effort made to practise health care. (One respondent did not answer the perceived effort made question. The chi square analyses that showed no significant correlation are indicated by 'n.s.'.)

arrangements and perceived health status. There is not a statistically significant correspondence between effort made and living arrangement. The respondents who were interviewed felt their health suffered as a result of losing their mother's care when they left the family home. The men felt as though their diet had deteriorated for lack of food preparation skills, and because they couldn't be bothered cooking, or did not know how to cook, healthy meals. Further, other than a family member who was a health-care professional, the mother was the only family member whom the respondents consulted when they received conflicting health care advice. A loss in overall household income may also be significant in the deterioration of the men's perceived health,[29] although there was no such correspondence in this study.

There is a statistically significant correlation between those who perceive the effort they make to keep healthy as low, and those who are willing to have sex where the risk of catching a sexually transmitted infection (STI) is high (Table 4). None of these men were interviewed and they offered little in the way of information in the questionnaire. However, the display of overt heterosexuality and power is inferred in some of the responses. Mr 55, for example, said that he would like to 'get a nice chick and just cane her'.

Youthline conducted a study to discuss issues of relationships, sex, and sexuality with seventy-five men and women of all ethnicities aged fifteen to twenty years.[30] While there was a general awareness of the health risks of unprotected sex with a partner of unknown STI status among the respondents to this study and those who use Youthline's services, it appears that the pursuit of pleasure is prioritised for some men over caring for their sexual health. Few men in the Youthline study were concerned about getting a woman pregnant, whereas there was widespread concern about contracting an STI. 'The women felt that for men their top priorities were the selfish pursuit of pleasure and looking good in the eyes of their mates'.[31] A 'small' (unspecified) proportion of men replying to Youthline said they were prepared to have sex without a condom; 'some used to think it was pretty cool to have sex without a condom for enjoyment and [for this reason] it was great to get your girlfriend on the pill' (Pakeha, 17–18 years).[32] Further, a respondent to Youthline's study said, 'I found all my friends tried to project this image of a strong sort of heterosexuality and at an all guys school it generally makes them feel more secure; compensate by being extra masculine' (Pakeha, 19–20).[33]

Homophobia and sexual prudishness are problematic for sexual and reproductive health care. The response of the 'general public' to media personality Paul Holmes' frankness about his prostate cancer was the subject of a 'Dialogue' article in the *New Zealand Herald*.[34] The article accused the public of being 'hypocritical'. Its author says, 'Word on the street in smart parts of Auckland is that we've all heard more than enough about Holmes and his prostate cancer … It's ironic really because this is probably the same crowd that eagerly digested every last scrap of the Fleur Revell story. Back then, his sex life was a hot topic …'.[35] Mr 14, during his interview, discussed the need for greater awareness of the risk of prostate cancer. Alluding to the prudishness and homophobia in our society, he said:

> most guys I think wouldn't go anyway although for most of those a blood test is fine and it is only if the blood test turns out to be inconclusive that there is any need to have a ahhem (*clears his throat and laughs*), physical check (*laughs*) and it's the physical test which puts a lot of guys off I think, unless you are that way inclined …

Individuals who smoke tobacco and use illegal drugs are more likely to perceive their general health status to be low (Table 3). There is also a high correlation between perceived health status and effort made to look after one's health. However, there is not a significant correlation between perceiving the effort made to look after one's health as low, and smoking tobacco and using drugs. A possible reason for this will be discussed below.

Among the respondents to this study there is less agreement on what the health risks are with illegal drug use, or even if there are health risks. Nevertheless, the risks of engaging in illegal activity featured in the discussion. This reflects the emphasis of the government's activity regarding illegal drugs. Those who recognised their drug use as posing health risks (seven of nineteen users) again spoke of the benefits they gained from drug use as compensating for the risks. During the focus group, Mr 60 said that 'there's more violence and crime around this stuff [holding up a beer bottle], people getting lagered, becoming Mr Toughman trying to pick fights, whereas if you sit, have a joint, you're a bit more mellow, you tend to just want to sit and mellow out and wind down'. Mr 56 replied with 'until the cops come and bust ya'. Likewise, Mr 31 said, 'I don't think it is risky unless you do it in public places where cops may be lingering'.

There is no association between perceived effort made and perceived health status and alcohol use. However, drinking alcohol is spoken of in very much the same sense as tobacco and drugs – that is, in terms of allowing a release from stress and socio-economic pressures.

Discussion

Social Context and Health

The results of this study indicate the many ways in which masculinity and health interact in the lives of the respondents. Many issues have also been raised; for example the interplay between socio-economic realities and health, illness and health care. Many studies have demonstrated that socio-economic status is a major determinant of health status.[36] However, as we have seen, the sample group's perceived health status compares poorly to their demographic group as a whole, despite the sample group having a generally favourable socio-economic profile. Reasons for this incongruence may be found in the beliefs and behaviours of the sample group.

In practising health care, the respondents spoke of needing to strike a balance between the 'costs' of health care practice, lifestyle choice, identity, and socio-economic pressures. This can be interpreted as the respondents practising health care as they see fit according to their day-to-day concerns and the dynamics of the social setting. On occasion, health care would be abstained from or delayed if peer pressure, team commitments, employer demands, the need to study, or choice dictated that this be so. Some men felt that their peers and/or their role as an employee or sports team member (especially during competition) discouraged health care. As discussed earlier, young men's desire for, and limited claims to, manhood may make them particularly prone to social pressures that discourage health care.

Mr 3 referred to sometimes feeling peer pressure to opt for the unhealthy option:

Interviewer What about if you come across a situation where you've got to be either healthy or unhealthy, how do you decide what to do?

Mr 3 … well I don't know, it depends on the situation. Sometimes I couldn't give a crap and I would just do [the 'unhealthy' option], I mean I am more likely to probably go to, um, peer pressure if you would like to call it that and sit down and have a few beers and chips and what ever goes down when I am with my mates. Whereas if I wasn't with them I would probably not do that …

Nevertheless, friends were among the most trusted consultants when the men sought health care advice. 'Mother' was also important as a confident.

The respondents expressed a need to be able to trust both the validity of the information, and the person giving the care or advice.

Reasons for wanting to keep one's illness and injury to oneself or telling only one's trusted associates and friends are linked with the common perception of health care being expensive and culturally limited to Pakeha health practices. In addition, a man must enter a social engagement where his performance is converse to that validated by hegemonic structures of masculinity: that is, the demonstration of control, authority, toughness, stoicism, and ability. Exposing one's 'weakness' to another subordinates oneself in a relationship of unequal power. The loss of personal autonomy and authority that result from admitting a weakness to another may be crucial barriers to seeking health care advice from people whom the men do not personally know. For this reason, establishing a trusting relationship with health-care professionals is very important. A reluctance to seek advice often results in men waiting to see if they can cope with the negative effects of illness or injury, hoping that they will recover without taking time out from performing tasks required of them as men, or as a team member, provider, employee, or lover. These tasks are integral to masculine self-esteem. This may be the reason why professional care is more likely to be sought once the ability to perform such tasks becomes a problem.

The importance of social context is reflected in residential arrangements. As referred to earlier in this chapter, men who moved away from the family home felt, on average, that their health suffered. One reason for this perceived drop is gendered domestic roles. Respondents referred to their poor cooking abilities, not being interested in cooking, and Mum having the responsibility for the family's health care. A disruption of young people's social network, often a result of moving away from the family home, has also been associated with a perception of lower health status.[37] This may be a particularly important determinant of health for this age group, as young men and women sometimes move a long way from the family home, town, and friends with whom they grew up. Indeed, a respondent to this study, Mr 24, left home to live in another city upon graduation from university, and felt that his health suffered because the move disrupted his lifestyle.

Self-Reported Health Status

An important influence on the respondent's perception of his health status was his current lifestyle and what he wanted to do. Some men knew that certain behaviours affected their health negatively, but because the negative effects did not particularly bother them (for example, they were not having to provide for dependents, or even go to work the next day), less than ideal health was acceptable to them. Thus, the perception of health risk and status is dependent upon life course and social context.

Physical potential is very important in estimating both health status and masculinity. This is reflected in the men's concepts of 'health' being very physical and task-oriented, in addition to the newspaper data. In estimating their masculine capital and health status, men appear to be influenced by the activities that other men practise, compared to their own potential to practise those activities. However, chronic illness sufferers perceive themselves as not realistically being able to practise some activities and may exclude these from the ideal level they perceive themselves attaining. For example, Figure 2 shows that the haemophilia sufferers rated their health to be better on average than did the respondents to this study, but haemophilia sufferers and the writer's sample group have very different potentials for physical activity. Additionally, a school-aged boy with 'the invisible disability of severe haemophilia' was hassled by his mates for not playing rugby; in response to this he told his mother, 'I'd rather have my legs cut off so people could see it.'[38] If his legs were 'cut off' he believed his schoolmates could more readily see and understand his disability and would no longer hassle him for not playing rugby. Further, the disabled Paralympian Matt Slade said that he was 'disabled anyway' so he may as well run on his broken ankle.[39] As far as I am aware, the respondents to this study did not suffer from severe disabilities and may therefore have rated their own albeit unrealised physical potential and ideal health status with reference to élite athletes. Pakeha masculinities do not confer valuable cultural capital on male bodies and practices that cannot take heavy knocks or deliver massive amounts of power and stamina. The haemophilia sufferers' difficulties in developing a respected masculine identity are indicative of this.[40]

Concepts of Health and Healthy Practices

There is no correspondence between using drugs or tobacco, or being a heavy drinker and a perceived poor effort to practise health care. Those who perceived themselves as making a poor effort to practise health care were also likely to perceive themselves as having a poor health status (Figure 3). Yet, using illegal drugs and tobacco was associated with those who perceived themselves to have a poor health status (Table 3).

This finding points to Crawford's illustration of health as release.[41] Individuals who use illegal drugs and/or tobacco practise behaviours that are traditionally viewed as unhealthy, but these behaviours can be employed to provide a release from societal, mental and emotional pressure and can thereby be viewed as healthy. For example, those who recognised that their illegal drug use posed health risks (seven of nineteen users) spoke of the benefits of their drug use as partially, or totally, compensating for the health risks because it helped them to relax, unwind and have a good time. This may explain why the smokers and drug users did not necessarily see the effort they made to practise health care as low, but they did perceive their standard of health to be below average. For example, Mr 38, who also smokes tobacco, said, 'I know it is bad for me. I do it anyway because I enjoy smoking'. Crawford's[42] illustration of health as release may also explain why there is no statistically significant relationship between alcohol use, perceived health status, and the effort the men make to keep healthy.

For some of the respondents, demonstrating an ability to drink copious amounts of alcohol was a means of trying to claim masculine capital. One respondent said, '[I] used to get sick trying to prove I could drink more than I can' (Mr 44). Most drinkers said that they did not drink enough alcohol for their drinking to be a health risk. Many respondents would get sick 'most' times they drank alcohol but did not see their drinking as a health risk. The potentially adverse effects on their health may not be recognised for two reasons. First, because it helps to release stress, and secondly because heavy alcohol use is so ubiquitous among young men that its harmful effects are perceived by them as 'normal'. Hangovers, for example, are often referred to by the respondents as 'par for the course'.

The interplay between masculinities and alcohol, tobacco and illegal drug use, carries potentially positive as well as negative health consequences. The positive effects, however, are probably superficial and problematic. The respondents use alcohol and drugs as a coping mechanism where masculinity and other social structures appear to be a hindrance or, in other words, do not provide ready answers for coping with stress. A further relief from societal pressures may be found in Hodges' argument that alcohol provides some excuse for behaviours that do not conform to the standards of practice that apply when sober.[42]

Conclusions

Negotiation is required to strike a balance between health status, masculinity and the social setting, which on many occasions position masculinity and health care in conflict. Some of the respondents who reported low health status took illegal drugs, alcohol and tobacco, some of them lived away from the family home, and some of them made little effort to practise health care. Elite athletes, particularly the All Blacks, have been constructed as exemplars of masculinity in New Zealand, and they also influenced the respondents' conceptions of ideal health.

Between the dominant principles of masculinity and the construction of 'health for health's sake' as feminine, there is much to discourage men from practising health care. However, the gendered identity of health care is context dependent: practising health care is more acceptable to men when its purpose is to be healthy for the workplace, to enhance performance in a sporting capacity, to ensure one is able to provide for dependents, and to benefit one's intimate partner in a stable relationship. These social roles can encourage men to practise health care, but do not necessarily do so because the many confounding factors that exist in any one social setting complicate a linear response.

Overall, the concepts of health, illness and health care are fluid. They are difficult to isolate from day-to-day life, an individual's past, biological reality (such as degree of health, injury or illness), and his predictions of the future. Because of this, concepts of health, illness and health care cannot be explored in any detail without referring to the context in which individuals are discussing or experiencing them. Nevertheless, themes can be deduced from the study's data. First, the young men thought of an 'ideal' health status as one that facilitates the fulfilment of tasks; secondly, 'health' and 'illness' were for them largely physical concepts; and thirdly, men did 'not want to look feminine'.

It may be because masculinities can be undermined at any moment,[43] that many men prefer to squeeze the most out of themselves so that they continue to satisfy the demands of their role rather than accept a degree of incapacity when health problems arise. Demonstrating control over one's body is an immediately accessible medium for the demonstration of power and control which are valuable masculine qualities. Exaggeration of power and control over oneself may be particularly common practice among young men because they need to establish legitimate claims to adult manhood within a narrow hegemonic prescription, and in the end, hegemonic masculinity only makes sense in relation to people in positions of power recognising that one's actions are worthy of valuable masculine capital being conferred. In addition to socio-economic concerns of time and money, because health care practice is often constructed as a feminine practice, knowledge of the healthiest way in which to address a health concern does not always result in the healthiest option being practised by young men.

Acknowledgements

I would like to thank the following people and organisations for their assistance in the production of this work: firstly, the Health Research Council of New Zealand for granting me a Junior Health Award which has gone a long way towards meeting the research expenses of this work. Thanks also to the Anthropology Department at the University of Auckland, and in particular Dr Julie Park and Dr Judith Littleton, for continued support and advice, and to Jude McCool who kindly gave her own time to proofread and comment on earlier drafts of this work. Finally, thanks to my wife, Kathy Hood, who has helped with the production of this work in a number of ways and is the best partner one could hope for.

ten

Abducted by Aliens: Heterosexual men and sexual health

STEPHEN MCKERNON

Heterosexual men are omitted from specific analysis and discussion in sexual health policy. Silence about heterosexual male sexualities, including coercive and abusive practices, suggests difficulty in framing the issues afforded by heterosexual men within sexual health. Yet heterosexual men also have a significant share in the burden of sexually transmitted infections (STIs) in Aotearoa New Zealand. This chapter argues for improving sexual health in Aotearoa New Zealand by targeting heterosexual men and their sexual practices. Examples are given via studies in the promotion of condoms and provision of sexual health services to heterosexual men.[1]

The sexually transmitted infections gonorrhoea and chlamydia are increasing worldwide. Sexual health data in Aotearoa New Zealand indicate these STIs are most apparent among heterosexual men, and among young heterosexual Maori and Pacific Island men particularly.[2] Little is known about the relationship between heterosexual masculinities and STIs such as gonorrhoea or chlamydia, and as a result, opportunities for rapid and effective response to the current crisis are limited. Heterosexual masculinities and sexual practices are thus emerging as important sexual health issues in this country. There are also broader strategic opportunities for targeting heterosexual men: Hawkes and Hart suggest that emphasis on management of male sexual health may be more effective than approaches which often emphasise reproductive health, especially where resources are limited.[3] They emphasise that services targeting men need not detract from those for women and other groups.

This chapter discusses two qualitative research studies with male heterosexual clients of a sexual health service. The studies, which explored men's sexual health for the challenges posed to local masculinities, were undertaken within the established frameworks for sexual health in Aotearoa New Zealand, with the aim of progressing sexual health promotion and service delivery to heterosexual men. But issues raised by the men in these studies suggest opportunities outside the current framework for sexual health. The first section of this chapter discusses the recent position of heterosexual men in sexual health. The second section explores male heterosexual approaches to condom use and sexual health services. The position evolving from this work is that a powerful strategy for improving sexual health in Aotearoa New Zealand could involve targeting heterosexual men and their sexual practices specifically.

THE DISAPPEARANCE OF HETEROSEXUAL MEN FROM SEXUAL HEALTH

Sexually transmitted infections (STIs, formerly known as STDs and VDs) are known internationally as markers of poverty and marginalisation. The groups most at risk of STIs are identified as men who have sex with men, people living with HIV, indigenous peoples, youth, injecting drug users, sex workers and their clients, survivors of sexual abuse, people in prison and refugees.[4]

Some STIs have symptoms that are easily noticed and some do not. Holmes *et al.* indicate that STIs are more often asymptomatic (lacking symptoms) than symptomatic (having symptoms). Because of the asymptomatic bias in STIs, there is considerable opportunity for STI transmission by people who are unaware of their infection. Having said this, STIs in men are typically symptomatic, leading to easier detection, diagnosis and treatment. Sequelae (other health conditions) are also generally less severe in men, but significant problems including infertility and death still feature. The sequelae of STIs have the greater effects for women and reproductive health, though HIV/AIDS are also associated with more severe illnesses and death. In this context, sexual health in recent years has been strongly concerned with the burden of sexual infection for heterosexual women and for men who have sex with men.

Heterosexual men are omitted from specific attention in sexual health policy and service delivery. For example, local heterosexual masculinities are detailed in neither analyses of causal factors nor of strategic possibilities. In fact, heterosexuality and heterosexual men have not been a significant focus in research or policy internationally until very recently. For example, Holmes *et al.* discuss sexual practices among gay men and note the lack of corresponding analysis of 'heterosexual concomitants of particular sexual practices'.[5] This is not to say that heterosexual men are in any way a marginalised group. Rather, their position in sexual health is *unspecified* and is evaluated here with a view to influencing sexual health strategy.

There are three broad issues that influence evaluation of heterosexual men in sexual health strategy overall. These are (1) the impact heterosexual masculinities may have on the sexual health of men and their partners, (2) the limitation of exploratory discourses on male heterosexuality, and (3) statistics suggesting young heterosexual men bear a significant burden of sexual infection. These issues are discussed briefly below.

Heterosexual masculinities' impact on sexual health

Heterosexual masculinities and their sexual practices may influence the sexual health status of the community directly. Research on young male heterosexuals indicates sexual performance is a marker of maturity, and confers status in male heterosexual culture as proof of manhood.[6] The dominant male culture also constructs other performances as proofs. For example, drinking alcohol to excess is significant in local masculinities of all ages.[7] These studies of male cultures suggest that older or higher status male drinkers influence aspiring drinkers to behave in ways that confer such benefits as self-worth, a sense of belonging and a well-defined identity as a heterosexual male. But there is less understanding of more experienced men's influences on sexual practices of younger men. Heterosexual male sexual discourses seem largely oriented towards competing for status with male peers, one effect of which may be coercion of male peers into abusive sexual practices. But it is far from clear how local male cultures and their discourses impact on sexuality and sexual practices, how they contribute (negatively and positively) to men's sexual health, and how they might be influenced to do so in positive ways.

Having said this, some aspects of local male heterosexuality are well documented. For example, sexual coercion of women by male heterosexuals has been well documented in local research. A study by Gavey suggests 52 per cent of undergraduate women at an Auckland tertiary institution had experienced some form of coercion and 25 per cent had experiences of attempted or actual rape.[8] A national study of drinking practices shows that 27 per cent of women aged sixteen to twenty-four had been sexually harassed by heterosexual men, and 10 per cent of women had been harassed on at least five occasions in the last twelve months.[9] The sexual practices of local male heterosexuals must be understood in the context of local masculinities endorsing harm to women.

More recent work also suggests male heterosexual sexual practices are quite diverse,[10] even though their sexual discourses centre on vaginal penetration, and stigmatise practices such as anal sex. Studies of the incidence of heterosexual male anal sex (with women or men) suggest figures from about 7 per cent in Aotearoa New Zealand[11] to about 23 per cent among college students in a USA sample.[12] The latter study suggests use of condoms for heterosexual anal sex is lower than for vaginal sex. Halperin and Bailey claim that seven times more women engage in *unprotected* anal sex with men than men who have sex with men.[13] Local men's sexual practices may also impact in currently unrecognised ways.

The Ministry of Youth Affairs (MYA) is to be commended for developing a stance on the sexual health of young men specifically. The stance has been developed through analysis and strategy papers and research with Youthline.[14] Young men in the MYA/Youthline research consider their key issues are getting sex when they want, and managing their feelings about women and sex: 'The problem is girls and emotions'.[15] Young heterosexual men themselves articulate problems within local masculinities and their related sexual practices. Young men are 'naturally' supposed to want lots of sex, but the significance of this for sexual health strategy is easily overlooked. Existing evidence, fragmented as it is, suggests that local masculinities are problematic, impact directly within sexual health, and are open to influence both from without and within.

Heterosexual masculinity is not up for examination

Local heterosexual masculinities construct male heterosexuality as instinctual and requiring no explanation or exploration. As suggested, sex talk among heterosexual males is a public performance oriented towards having fun. Sensible discussion of sex and sexual practices may be ridiculed as effeminate, paranoid or overly serious. As a result, serious sex talk becomes stigmatised, and talk with close male friends proscribed by avoiding pressure or embarrassment. By comparison, sex talk with female partners is a marker of intimacy though men allocate the initiative to women.[16] Exploring significant issues within local male heterosexuality (such as the acceptance of the differing coercive practices with male friends and female partners) may be curbed by male resistance, by a broader complicity with inarticulate masculinity, or perhaps by the belief that the issues are simply too difficult to approach.

As a case in point, secondary school education offers a significant opportunity to generate discussion about and influence local male sexual discourses and practices. Some educators are careful to position sex within discussion of values and skills for relationships and casual sex, and in relation to socialising, gender identities and sexual practices. Discussion topics may include alcohol use, masturbation, stigmatising, peer pressure, sexual orientation, coercion and abuse, sexual pleasure, safer sex and self-esteem. For example, the Auckland Sexual Health Service has evolved and operated a successful peer sexuality support training programme covering such topics in Auckland schools for a number of years.

But sexuality education is the only topic in the curriculum requiring specific inclusion by the board of trustees. Education Review Office checks on sex education in schools in 1996 suggest only half of schools have completed the initial mandated consultation step, and very few offer the suggested target fourteen hours of sexuality education per pupil per school year.[17] Elliott notes the broad emphasis on biology and sex (as opposed to sexuality) and also notes the steady decrease in any sexuality education after the third form. By the seventh form any educational influences on male heterosexuality and its sexual practices are minimal.[18]

Examining male heterosexuality has not been a strength of sexual health policy strategy to date. Putting male heterosexuality up for examination by peers and within sexuality education is consistent with sexual health strategy targeting the young – and young men especially. The broader issue is generating differing discourses about local masculinities and their sexual practices, be it among teachers, boards or parents.

Heterosexual men are significant in STI statistics

Heterosexual men are significant in STIs statistics in Aotearoa New Zealand. The Institute of Environmental and Scientific Research (ESR) has provided statistics on STIs diagnosed in Aotearoa New Zealand for a number of years now. Contributing to the data by varying degrees are sexual health, family planning and student and youth health services.[19]

ESR data indicates that in 1999 about 36,000 people enquired about sexual health issues and 7,800 were diagnosed with STIs. About 96 per cent were diagnosed through sexual health services specifically, and in this data the Auckland Sexual Health Service (ASHS) alone diagnosed about 28 per cent of STI cases. The ESR data show that about half (45 per cent) of clients visiting sexual health services were men. Sexual orientation is not recorded in the data (so some are men having sex with men), but ASHS anecdotal information suggests about 80 per cent or more were men having sex with women (whether identifying as heterosexual or gay).

In ESR's data for sexual health services specifically, men are almost twice as likely as women to be diagnosed with an STI (though more women present at these services than men). About one in every seven European male clients had an STI: the figure is about one in every four for Maori or Pacific Island male clients. By comparison, about one in every thirteen European female clients had an STI, while the figure is about one in seven for Maori or Pacific Island female clients. This suggests the burden of infection is actually greater for men than for women, though STIs can be more difficult to diagnose in women, who may also be using other health services (such as family planning) for sexual health care.

The data does suggest that heterosexual men have a high, though different, burden of infection and a significant role in sexual health. Managing male heterosexual contributions to transmission of STIs can have a significant impact on sexual health more generally.

This section has suggested that local masculinities and their favoured sexual practices are profoundly implicated in the sexual health status of the community, and while there are significant gaps in understanding, this would point to targeting male heterosexuals specifically as a key group. Yet heterosexual men seem to have disappeared from sexual health policy and strategy, both in analysis of issues and in articulation of appropriate strategies.

THE REAPPEARANCE OF HETEROSEXUAL MEN IN SEXUAL HEALTH

Heterosexual men reappear in sexual health largely in relation to promotion and use of condoms. As a result, much attention has centred on overcoming men's resistances to condom use.

Heterosexual men reappear in sexual health in promotional contexts and alongside discourses of responsibility. Hawkes and Hart note that discourses of 'responsibility' in sexual and reproductive health are linked with heterosexual men ('rights' are linked with heterosexual women).[20] This may be what Ministry of Health documents are heading towards in 'promoting responsible sexual behaviour' to address unwanted pregnancy, HIV/AIDS and STDs collectively.[21] Ethical references in relation to gender identities or sexual practices in sexual health discourse are otherwise rare. In fact, unprotected and unsafe sex may be considered the norm among heterosexuals in Aotearoa New Zealand. Heterosexual values for romance, love and family mean that unprotected sex is linked to trust, intimacy, maturity and procreative sex.

Condoms are recognised as an effective physical barrier to both STIs and conception and are promoted internationally in sexual and reproductive health programmes. Condoms have had broad success and their use may now be linked with age cohorts in Aotearoa New Zealand,[22] though there may also be variations in contraceptive and regional use.[23] In sexual health promotions through public media, condoms have the incidental advantage of implying caution with diverse sexual practices without having to specify them.

But where sexual health emphasises women's sexual and reproductive health, condom use might seem to be a woman's responsibility. Gavey and McPhillips note condom promotions are increasingly targeting heterosexual women, though women may find it difficult to require or negotiate condom use successfully.[24] A broad emphasis on promoting condoms to heterosexual men may seem surprising where sexual health policy omits analysis of local heterosexual masculinities and provides no clear strategic rationale. Promoting condoms also seems tangential to more important issues, such as managing coercive practices among heterosexual men. Where local masculinities place value on sexual performance as a marker of masculinity, the condom's barriers to performance and satisfaction might also shape its use within sexual health strategy. It may seem surprising that condoms are given such strategic prominence and that heterosexual men use them at all, but they are and they do.

LOCAL MEN AND THE TOTAL CONDOM USER

In 1996 the Auckland Sexual Health Service (ASH) developed a study of condom use among male heterosexual clients of the service.[25] Of particular interest was how heterosexual men constructed their 'own' condom use and non-use in relation to masculinity, to sexual partners, to STIs and to sexual health messages.

Individual interviews with eleven male heterosexual clients used unstructured questioning and discussion to explore the issues. The individual interview was chosen to fit with a broad emphasis on anonymity and confidentiality in sexual health. Understandings gained from each interview were transferred to discussion in the next, so the small number of interviews could be used to generate important insights. An important step in interview design was the decision to take a stand in favour of condom use where this would contribute to understanding the men's concerns. All interviews were tape-recorded and transcripts were read and analysed using discourse analytic methods. The study was approved by the Health Ethics Committee of the time. A recent review of the transcripts has also assisted in providing this account. The men ranged in age from late teens to mid-forties and identified as Pakeha, though one also identified as Samoan. The men varied in their reasons for presenting at the service and taking part in the study: some had visited the service with questions only, while others had sought help with STIs and issues with sex. Overall they were grateful to ASH and wanted to contribute something in return. A particular issue in analysis and reporting was the diversity of attitudes the men had in relation to condom use and non-use.

These men said discussion of sexuality, risks and condom use was gendered and varied according to the context of use. For example, men said they might stay silent or joke about sex with male peers to avoid being ridiculed and portrayed as effeminate, weak or overly serious. Sexist humour and competitive talk about sex, for example, were primarily directed at other males. There was an implicit emphasis on successful performance, such as when telling sex jokes, as a generic way of fitting in with a male peer group.

> I mean it's … sex is still a point of embarrassment for some, or most, I don't know. Especially talking about condom use, never hear it. Yeah, serious with your mates is very rare, I'd say. Very, very rare. Unless you're talking, you know, unless something happened, like a funeral or whatever … even then I don't know how to talk to the, oh, father about having his new [unplanned] kid. Never, yeah, the odd time I have talked seriously to a couple of my mates, you know, but they try to avoid it, I'd say, most of the time. They ah, they know how to get around it, change the subject, or ignore you, or call you a flossie or whatever … tell you to fuck off, yeah, blouse. (5, Pakeha, 1996)

For these men, sexual discourses with partners emphasised sensitivity and intimacy. The man's honesty marked out his seriousness about the relationship, and naked (condom-less) sex marked out mutual trust and intimacy. The man's concern with 'making her come' was one way of constructing male sensitivity and intimacy. Negotiating condom use was marked by an apparently pro-feminist discourse (women are in charge of their own bodies), in which it was then up to the woman to decide on ('enforce') condom use for her own reasons.

Men discursively constructed sexual safety as parallel to safety concerns in manual and trades work. Condoms were compared to seatbelts, work boots and helmets: these protect the wearer only from external harms (though condoms aim to protect both partners). The ethical framework for condoms was protecting the heterosexual male user from the risks assumed in a woman partner. As a result, deciding on condom use was founded in notions of risk from women, while also allocating sexual health decisions to women. In local masculinities, men may not take the initiative and if women insist, men may still resist.

Using condoms was also modified by the centrality of 'protecting his masculine image'. This typically meant not using condoms because it was unmanly. But in one example, a man argued that because he rejected rugby-and-beer Kiwi blokes and was known to be effeminate, he didn't need to use condoms – he wasn't a threat to women.

Condoms were understood as a barrier to STIs and pregnancy, but more importantly, were also experienced as a barrier to pleasure and emotional intimacy. Condoms were favoured with casual and short-term partners where protection was needed, and trust was less important. If the partnership lasted, increasing intimacy and trust led to reduced use of condoms against STIs, and switching to non-barrier methods of contraception. At this time both partners were at risk of STI transmission. Condoms were associated with less mature sexualities and/or at an extreme, with sexual promiscuity. These findings are supported by a larger quantitative study by Barry *et al.*[26]

Peterman *et al.* summarise the relationship of condom use with sexual practice as 'safe sex with risky partners and risky sex with safe partners'.[27] To impact fully on STI prevalence, correct and consistent condom use must occur, especially among people who are highly sexually active. But, for example, men in the study said they might put on a condom after genital contact during foreplay (incorrect use) or with most but not all casual partners (inconsistent use), and not with regular partners (where other forms of contraception were being used).

Mixing condoms and heterosexual men raises important issues within sexual health. First, condom promotions have emphasised sex practices: this affords men the luxury of resisting 'unmanly' condom use from within the dominant masculinity. Second, sexual health has relied on promoting condom use as a key strategy, though this alone is inadequate for managing the risks afforded by heterosexual men. Finally, attention to the masculinities and/or the sexualities themselves might offer more powerful strategies. For example, some condom manufacturers have shifted their emphasis away from safer sex to sensuality and pleasure.[28]

In the ASH study above, the challenge was to construct a masculinity fitting with correct, consistent, complete use of condoms among sexually active heterosexual males (some diagnosed with STIs). This task was explored during interviews and the requisite condom use was described as 'always, from start to finish, no exceptions'. It is called 'total condom use' here for brevity and to signal key issues.

First, the men generally positioned the total condom user as paranoid, immature or calculating. Paranoia was linked with not being able to trust a female partner, immaturity with youthful sexual activities and calculated use with the early phase of a relationship. The prospect of total condom use represented a severe curtailment of male heterosexual sexuality. Second, some men positioned total condom use as very sophisticated. In context it is important to note that some men were dissatisfied with their experiences of masculinity and others were forced to assess theirs because they had an STI. The possibility of total condom use suggested a shift to a condom-based masculinity and/or sexuality (while the penis was still the centre of attention).

The total condom user was constructed as an appealing alternative to the generic beer-oriented local male heterosexual and his typical sexual practices. The user was variously described as confident, respectful, responsible, sexy and sensual, trustworthy, mature, articulate, skilled in relationships, sophisticated, fun-loving, placing less emphasis on getting sex, self-disciplined in condom use and knowing how to have a great time with women. It was difficult to identify examples of local masculinities or real men who fitted this profile. On the other hand, one man commented that men usually prefer to see themselves this way anyway.

A study by Bryan, Aiken and West suggests women like men more when men take the initiative to discuss and request condom use.[29] But women may also feel this diminished romance and excitement, and men fear this diminishes their chances of getting sex. Generating an appealing local masculinity oriented to managing these issues seems a viable and valuable approach.

Men in the ASH study suggested promoting condoms using the shock-tactics approach of television campaigns against local masculinities, such as those for 'drinking and driving' and domestic violence. Within the same framework, others suggested creating 'condom coaches' – men who made sure mates were safe (like non-drinking drivers). Others suggested humorous condom advertisements on TV or dramatising safer sex issues through television programmes such as *Shortland Street*. These were generally measures to build condom-loving discourses and condom-oriented heterosexual male cultures.

The total condom user did not represent a major shift in masculinity overall. But he did suggest a discernible gap, an aspiration arising from dissatisfaction with local masculinities, and a corresponding attempt to construct a form of masculinity specifically addressing transmission of STIs. In the context of sexual health strategies the total condom user also represents a number of important shifts. First, he targets and appeals to heterosexual men specifically.

Second, he does not represent a didactic approach to condom promotions: rather, his power lies in his emotive appeal over other local masculinities. Third, the user neatly encapsulates the point of other safer sex practices. And finally, the user takes a stand against commercial production of car- and beer-oriented masculinities.

Generating male heterosexual sexual health

The Auckland Sexual Health Service explored sexual health and sexual health service issues for eighteen heterosexual men over the summer months of 1999-2000.[30] Similar studies have been conducted in Australia and suggest the services heterosexual men want have distinct profiles according to local masculinities.[31]

A qualitative method was employed to first develop a basic understanding of sexual health for local heterosexual men and then to design service components consistent with this. Individual interviews were the key method used: other formats were offered to men but were rejected through fears over lack of anonymity and confidentiality. In some cases other formats were used where men preferred a specific location (such as home) or chose to bring friends to the interview. The eighteen men ranged in STI status (some diagnosed as positive, others as negative) and age. Reweti Te Mete interviewed ten Maori men, and Stephen McKernon interviewed eight Pakeha men. The study was approved by the Health Ethics Committee of the time. Interviews were transcribed and translated for reading and analysis.

Foremost among the issues for heterosexual men was the broad stigmatising of sex, STIs and sexual health. Heterosexual discourses of contamination and protection and heterosexual homophobia are well documented in sexual health.[32] Mortensen details other effects stigma generates within sexual health services.[33]

The effect for male heterosexual men was to generate significant shame, whakama, fear and sometimes anger in relation to STIs and sexual health services. The men said they arrived at sexual health services in states of anxiety generated by stigma, exacerbated by mates' tales of service equipment and amplified by fear of death from HIV/AIDS. The shame and fear is significant enough to result in delays in presenting or failing to attend appointments, and the delay itself contributes to STI prevalence.[34]

Men also become preoccupied with scenarios such as having an 'umbrella' shoved down their penis (a mythical procedure), meeting a friend or seeing a sexual contact at the service, being propositioned by a gay client, getting an erection during the consultation, and being examined by a beautiful female clinician. Men's accounts indicated the service visit was usually the first time they had talked frankly about sexual practices, had their penis touched by anyone other than a mother or girlfriend, and had to reflect on 'their' sexual practices. The broad theme was feeling completely alienated from things masculine (hence the title of this chapter):

> There's an element of the only way of dealing with HIV positive and getting a test for AIDS, you know, is to make a joke about it ... he [his mate] made a joke about me being *abducted by aliens*, because that's the sort of thing they'd do. (1, Pakeha, 2000)

Another aspect was being stigmatised and treated as an alien. In the quote below, this is confirmed by a Maori man's experience of service at the main hospital reception:

> The nurses at the hospital reception just stared at me as if I was an *alien* or something. I thought of all places, I wouldn't get that prejudice at a hospital. (16, Maori, 2000)

Men diagnosed with an STI feared 'the end of sex' and no longer being a man. Over time these men sought ways of rebuilding their self-esteem and reconstructing masculinity around the stigma of having an STI, having safe sex only, living with a secret and communicating the issues with partners. Stigma and fears also shaped men's expectations of the service. Some expected professional, impersonal and purely medical procedures such as a blood test and a brief physical examination from a white-coated clinician. One metaphor for this was the warrant of fitness check for private vehicles – an expert checks the machine and signs a certificate to verify its roadworthiness: no questions are to be asked about the driver, his history or his recent practices.

Men's anxiety also impacted on their compliance with service staff (and with medications later) and on their ability to retain information. For example, some men had difficulty being completely honest about recent sexual practices and some could not remember seeing posters on the walls or hearing the clinician offer safe sex advice. The men generally constructed their relationships with sexual health services through metaphors of institutional authority: facing school teachers (for the younger man), employers and court judges. In their accounts, the men positioned themselves as powerless, vulnerable, alienated and struggling to hold their own. They identified with terrified boys on their first day at school, anxious men attending job interviews and depressed men facing charges at court. The ethic was again uni-directional: sexual health was being done to them and they were only there because they had to be.

> I've no regrets, and only disappointments. Especially having to make this appointment. (Graffiti board in men's waiting room, ASH offices)

Some were more confident of their relationship with the service (especially returning clients). Some had positioned condom use, regular sex check-ups, prompt use of the service if symptoms were noticed and a comfortable relationship overall within a more sophisticated masculinity, subsequently referred to as the effective service user. An overwhelming concern among the men was to preserve anonymity and confidentiality as a client of the service, and to be treated by non-judgemental service staff. They said overall the visit to the sexual health service was a traumatic experience, and they expressed gratitude for the professional, friendly, direct and non-judgemental approach of service staff. Talking about these aspects of the visit with close male friends was common.

Overall the men wanted specific information on sex and STIs for adult men. This was underpinned by shame about being an adult man with serious questions about sex and by reluctance to have 'adult sex education classes' in public and/or with other men. Remote access technologies (phone, Internet, print media, TV) were preferred because they could be used from home and did not place men at risk of identification or shame. Men wanted to peruse the issues in anonymous and impersonal ways, such as seeing them dramatised on *Shortland Street*.

Men also requested specific service components. For example, Maori men requested services oriented towards Maori, including Maori language and staff. Some suggested a self-examination guide for penis and testes, information and advice from sexual health service clinicians, mobile services, and having a liaison person within the service who could provide more general sexual health information and advice.

These ideas and requests suggest two important tasks. First, while anonymous, confidential and non-judgemental service was the preferred approach to sexual health, this also preserved silence around heterosexual masculinity and men's sexual practices. Public discussion of the issues and destigmatising of sex, STIs and/or sexual health services for male heterosexuals is an important task. Accounting for the *sexual* in sexual health must remain central. Second, a related task is building sensible heterosexual male sexual discourses to address tasks such as blocking coercive practices (among male peers and with women) and building respect for sexual health.

Local masculinities: Not really abducted, but not fully sexual

This chapter argues for improving sexual health in Aotearoa New Zealand by targeting heterosexual men and their sexual practices. The studies suggest that heterosexual men feel sex is so stigmatised that as adults they find themselves needing information and advice on sexual health matters. Some nurture an investment in shifting local masculinities and sexual practices for themselves. It appears that different approaches to the provision of sexual health services and to promotion of condoms may have effects beyond the domain of sexual health.

Following Connell, it seems important to avoid reifying a hegemonic masculinity or positioning local masculinities as uniformly bad or unchangeable.[35] The incremental shifts in condom use promotions and sexual health services suggested above may raise issues over complicity with, or within a hegemonic masculinity. In context, it seems important to acknowledge existing complicities as well as anticipating potential ones. The chapter emphasises that improved management of heterosexual male sexuality may be a powerful strategy in sexual health.

About the Authors

R.W. CONNELL

Louisa Allen currently lectures within the School of Education and Institute for Research on Gender at the University of Auckland. The research upon which the chapter in this book is based formed part of her doctorate undertaken at the University of Cambridge, and was made possible by the support of a postgraduate scholarship from the Health Research Council of New Zealand. At the end of her current lecturing contract she will take up a postdoctoral fellowship from the Foundation for Research Science and Technology in order to use her doctoral findings to design a sexuality education programme for students in their last two years of secondary schooling.

Clive Aspin (Ngati Maru ki Hauraki) has recently received his PhD in public health and is based in Sydney where he is the programme manager of an education programme for people who inject drugs. He has worked for many years in the field of HIV/AIDS as a community worker, policy analyst, lecturer and researcher. His research interests include gay men's sexuality, migration, identity and indigenous health issues. He has a strong interest in trans-Tasman migration and the effects of this on gay Maori men during the time of the AIDS epidemic. He lives in Sydney with his partner, Terry, and their son, Louis Manu-o-te-Rangi.

Bob Connell is Professor of Education at the University of Sydney, and was formerly Professor of Sociology at the University of California, Santa Cruz (1992–95), Professor of Australian Studies at Harvard University (1991–92), and Professor of Sociology, Macquarie University, Sydney (1976–91). Born 1944 in Sydney, Australia, he has a BA in history and psychology from the University of Melbourne and a PhD in government from the University of Sydney. He is author or co-author of sixteen books, including *Class Structure in Australian History, Making the Difference, Gender and Power, Schools and Social Justice, Masculinities* and *The Men and the Boys*. He is a past-president of the Sociological Association of Australia and New Zealand, a member of a range of policy advisory committees, and a contributor to research journals in sociology, education, political science, gender studies and related fields. His current research concerns are gender equity, globalisation and intellectuals.

Stephen McKernon MA, MSc has worked as a qualitative market researcher for the past decade across most industries, specialising in brand development for local and international companies. He has an MA in English and an MSc in psychology and currently works with QZONE, New Zealand's only specialist qualitative marketing and research company. He is interested in sexual health centres, and in finding practical ways to influence coercion within local male heterosexual sexual identities and practices. He is also interested in theorising a postmodern qualitative research in the marketing context.

Anthony O'Connor has an MA(Hons) in anthropology from the University of Auckland. He is interested in gender and health. Tony works with a team at the Mental Health Foundation in Auckland who are developing and facilitating a peer support group that aims to help individuals improve their quality of life. He is also preparing for PhD study in the field of medical anthropology, focusing on stress-related illness and how people cope with it. He lives in Auckland, is happily married to Kathy, and is always planning his next overseas trip.

Terry O'Neill has a PhD from the Queen's University of Belfast's School of Sociology and Social Policy and is the Co-ordinator for Students and Staff with Disabilities at the University of Auckland. His central research interest is the constitution of masculinities and their relationship to the formulation and management of multiple male identities in contemporary social settings.

Anna Paris MA (Hons) Sociology, University of Auckland, is research assistant for the Institute for Research on Gender at the University of Auckland. She is also working on her PhD thesis in sociology, exploring some of the meanings that emerge when poststructural and postmodern feminist discourses are applied to the cosmetically enhanced female body. Her other interests include post-human theories of the body, studies on gender and sexualities, and the cultural construction of pathologised bodies.

Julie Park, Tamasailau Suaalii-Sauni, Melani Anae, and **Ieti Lima** are all postgraduate students or staff members in anthropology, sociology and Pacific studies at the University of Auckland. Their research interests and publications include gender, Pacific identities and cultures, Aotearoa New Zealand society, health and health policy, and research methods. **Nite Fuamatu** works for the Accident Compensation Corporation (ACC) on Pacific issues in Wellington, and **Kirk Mariner** works in health promotion for Pacific peoples in Auckland.

Richard Pringle is a lecturer in the Department of Leisure Studies at the University of Waikato, where he teaches undergraduate papers in sport sociology and pedagogy, and a graduate paper on research philosophies. His doctoral research uses a post-structuralist approach to help understand how the experience of injury and pain, for males who have played rugby union, both challenges and reinforces dominating discourses of manliness. In his non-work time Richard enjoys sharing the care of his young sons with his marriage partner, Dixie, trips to the beach, cooking, listening to an eclectic mix of music and the occasional social game of tennis or volleyball.

Heather Worth is Senior Research Fellow and Deputy Director of the Institute for Research on Gender at the University of Auckland, has a PhD from the University of Auckland and is New Zealand's leading social researcher in the area of HIV and AIDS. She has been involved in sexuality and gender research for the last eight years. She has published extensively in international journals and has written two books, *Derrida Downunder* (2001) and *Reckless Vectors: AIDS and Criminality* (forthcoming).

Notes

Introduction

1. R.W. Connell (1995). *Masculinities* (Berkeley: University of California Press).
2. Ibid., p. 67.
3. Ibid., p. 71.
4. G.L. Mosse (1996). *The Image of Man: The Creation of Modern Masculinity* (New York and Oxford: Oxford University Press), introduction.
5. R.W. Connell (1995), p. 3.
6. Ibid., p. 52.
7. J. Phillips (1996 revised edition). *A Man's Country? The Image of the Pakeha Male – A History* (New Zealand: Penguin Books), p. 86.
8. See J. Butler (1990). *Gender Trouble: Feminism and the Subversion of Identity* (New York and London: Routledge); E. Grosz (1994). *Volatile Bodies: Towards a Corporeal Feminism* (Bloomington: Indiana University Press); M. Foucault (1978). *The History of Sexuality: An Introduction* (Trans. by R. Hurley) (New York: Pantheon).
9. J. Butler (1990), p. 6.
10. J. Allen (ed.) (1996). Growing up Gay: New Zealand men tell their stories (Auckland: Godwit); P. Wells and R. Pilgrim (eds) (1997). *Best Mates: Gay Writing in Aotearoa New Zealand* (Auckland: Reed)
11. For example, S. Frosh (1994). *Sexual Difference: Masculinity and Psychoanalysis* (London and New York: Routledge); G.I. Fogel, F.M. Lane and R.S. Liebert (eds) (1986). *The Psychology of Men: New Psychoanalytic Perspectives* (New York: Basic Books).
12. For example, R.W. Connell (1995); J. Weeks (2000). *Making Sexual History* (Malden, Mass: Polity Press); V. Seidler (1989). *Rediscovering Masculinity: Reason, Language and Sexuality* (London, New York: Routledge).
13. See M. Foucault (1978). *The History of Sexuality* (trans. R. Hurley) (London: Penguin).
14. Ibid.
15. J. Phillips, (1996), pp. 26–7.
16. S. Eldred-Grigg (1984). *Pleasures of the Flesh: Sex and Drugs in Colonial New Zealand, 1840–1915* (Wellington: Reed).
17. J. Phillips (1987).
18. Ibid., p. 70.

19 Cited in J. Phillips (1987), p. 188.
20 Ibid., p. 169.
21 M. Foucault (1990), p. 141.
22 J. Phillips (1987), p. 242.
23 Report of the Committee of the Board of Health into Venereal Disease in New Zealand (AJHR) (1922), H-3A, p.21
24 M. Foucault, (1990), pp. 32–33.
25 Cited in J. Phillips (1987), p. 100.
26 T. King (1906). *The Evils of Cram* (Dunedin: Whitcombe & Tombs), p. 27.
27 L. Star (1999). 'New Masculinities Theory: Post Structuralism and Beyond', in R. Law, H. Campbell and J. Dolan (eds), *Masculinities in Aotearoa/New Zealand* (Palmerston North: Dunmore), p. 243.
28 D. Brown (1997). 'Spilling the Beans', in P. Wells and R. Pilgrim (eds), *Best Mates: Gay Writing in Aotearoa New Zealand* (Auckland: Reed), p. 81.
29 L. Star, (1992). 'Undying Love, Resisting Pleasures: Women Watch Telerugby', in R. du Plessis (ed.), *Feminist Voices: Women's Studies Texts for Aotearoa/New Zealand* (Auckland: Oxford University Press), p. 133.
30 M. Foucault (1990), p. 44.
31 L. Star. 'Wild Pleasures: Watching Men on Television', *Women's Studies Journal* 10 (1) (1994), pp. 27–57.
32 M. King (ed.) (1988). *One of the Boys: Changing Views of Masculinity in New Zealand* (Auckland: Heinemann), pp. 149–150.
33 M. Foucault (1984). 'On the Genealogy of Ethics: An Overview of Work in Progress' in P. Robinson (ed.), *The Foucault Reader* (Middlesex: Penguin), p. 372.
34 K. Ireland, (1988). 'One of the Bohemians', in M. King (ed.), *One of the Boys: Changing Views of Masculinity in New Zealand* (Auckland: Heinemann), p. 101.
35 M. King (1987), p. 150.
36 J. Phillips (1987), pp. 219–220.
37 See M. Foucault (1990), p. 35.
38 S. Hunt (1996). 'Sam Hunt', in Jim Sullivan, *Catholic Boys: New Zealand Men Talk to Jim Sullivan* (Auckland: Penguin), p. 38.
39 G. McGee (1998). 'Sweet Bird' in M. King (ed.), p. 157.
40 J. McNab (1993). *A Social and Historical Overview: Male Homosexuality in New Zealand* (submitted in partial fulfilment of a Master of Arts Sociology, University of Auckland), p. 214.
41 See P. Wells and R. Pilgrim, (1997).
42 Ibid., p. 10.
43 See J. McNab (1993).
44 M. Foucault (1990), p. 49.
45 J. Ferguson (1949). 'A Study of Six Boys Involved with Homosexuals', *NZ Science Review* 7 (5) (May), pp. 70–2; see also B. James (1967a). 'Behaviour Therapy Applied to Homosexuality', *NZ Medical Journal* 66 (423), pp. 752–4 and B. James (1967b). 'Learning therapy and homosexuality', *NZ Medical Journal* 66 (423), pp. 748–51.
46 B. Logan (1988), p. 206.
47 A. Sharp (1994). *Leap into the Dark: The Changing Role of the State in New Zealand since 1984* (Auckland: Auckland University Press).
48 J. McNab and H. Worth (1998), p. 6.

49 M. Foucault (1990), p. 44

50 M. Mac an Ghaill (1994). *The Making of Men: Masculinities, Sexualities and Schooling* (Buckingham: Open University Press).

51 Historically HIV has predominately affected adult men in New Zealand. Of the 1478 people diagnosed with HIV by the end of 2000, 86 per cent were male (AIDS New Zealand, 2000). An estimated 80 per cent of that group comprised of men who have sex with other men

52 H. Worth (1996). 'Men who have Sex with Men: Sexual Patterns in New Zealand' in P. Davis (ed.), *Intimate Details and Vital Statistics: AIDS, Sexuality and the Social Order in New Zealand* (Auckland: Auckland University Press); S. Rosser (1991). *Male Homosexual Behaviour and the Effect of AIDS Education: a Study of Behaviour and Safer Sex in New Zealand and South Australia* (New York: Praeger).

53 M. Kimmel and M. Messner (1989). *Men's Lives* (New York: MacMillan); C. Waldby, S. Kippax and J. Crawford, 'Research Note: Heterosexual Men and "Safe Sex" Practice', *Sociology of Health and Illness* 15 (2) (1993), pp. 246–256.

54 Prostate cancer was the leading male site for cancer registrations in 1995. This rate has almost trebled since 1990 and this can be partly attributed to changes in cancer diagnosis and reporting. New Zealand has the third highest mortality rate for prostate cancer amongst OECD countries. (Ministry of Health, 1999a).

55 J. Phillips (1996), p. 121.

56 R. Kirby, M. Kirby and R. Farah (1999). *Men's Health: Closing the Gender Gap* (Oxford: Isis Medical Media Limited); T. O'Dowd and D. Jewell (eds), (1998). *Men's Health* (Oxford: Oxford University Press).

57 Ministry of Health, (1999), p. 14. Boys also have a higher death rate than girls during the first year of life (7.2 male deaths per 1,000 live births compared with 6.3 female deaths per 1,000 births in 1995–1997) (Statistics New Zealand (1999), p. 26.

58 P. Van Buynder and J. Smith. 'Mortality, Myth or Mateship Gone Mad: the Crisis in Men's Health', *Health Promotion Journal of Australia* 5 (3) (1995), p. 9.

59 A. Zodgerkar, (1999). 'The "Greying" of New Zealand', in P. Davies and K. Dew (eds), *Health and Society in Aotearoa/New Zealand.* (Oxford: Oxford University Press), p. 97.

60 North Health (1996). *The Health of Men – A Discussion Document* (Auckland: North Health), p. 4.

61 These include:

- Tobacco consumption (except in the 15-24 age group)
- Alcohol consumption

The areas of concern for men's health highlighted in the North Health study were:

- Being overweight but not obese
- Death by homicide
- First admissions to mental health services (except age 65–74)
- Higher asthma deaths in the elderly.

62 Statistics New Zealand (2000), p. 202.

63 However, it is also possible to point to areas in which women experience health disadvantages. For instance, registration rates in 1995 for cancer of the colon (15–64 years), pancreas (65 years plus) and skin melanoma (15–44 years) were all higher for women (Ministry of Health, 1999, p. 215). The 1996/97 disability survey also indicates that more women have disabilities (with females representing 54.3

per cent of all adults with a disability) (Statistics New Zealand. (1999) *New Zealand Now: Women* (1998 edition) Wellington: Statistics New Zealand, p. 28). Although females live longer than males, males self report better health-related quality of life (Ministry of Health, 1999, p. 21) Similarly, smoking-related diseases, including chronic obstructive respiratory disease and lung cancer, are declining among males, but not yet among females (Ministry of Health, 1999, p. 6).

64 Statistics New Zealand (2000), p. 195.

65 R. Connell (2000). *The Men and the Boys* (Sydney: Allen and Unwin), p. 181.

66 North Health (1996), p. 2.

67 Ministry of Health (1999). *Our Health, Our Future: The Health of New Zealanders* (Wellington: New Zealand Ministry of Health), p. 14.

68 Ibid., p. 15.

69 J. Watson (2000). *Male Bodies: Health, Culture and Identity* (Buckingham: Open University Press), p. 75.

70 Statistics New Zealand (2000), p. 179.

71 Statistics New Zealand (1998). *New Zealand Now: Young New Zealanders* (1998 Edition) (Wellington: Statistics New Zealand), p. 85.

72 R. Connell (2000); M.C. Robertson (1994) *Unruly Sites: Subjectivity and Masculine Enfleshment.* Thesis submitted in partial fulfilment of Master of Arts (Department of Psychology, University of Auckland); T. Jefferson, 'Muscle, 'Hard Men' and 'Iron' Mike Tyson: Reflections on Desire, Anxiety and the Embodiment of Masculinity', *Body and Society* 4 (1) (1998), pp. 77–98, J. Watson (2000).

73 A. Parker (1996). 'Sporting Masculinities: Gender Relations and the Body', in M. Mac an Ghail (ed.), *Understanding Masculinities* (Buckingham: Open University Press); R. Majors (1990). 'Cool Pose: Black Masculinity and Sports', in M. Messner and D. Sabo (eds), *Sport, Men and the Gender Order* (Champaign: Human Kinetics); S. Gilroy, 'The EmBody-ment of Power: Gender and Physical Activity', *Leisure Studies* 8 (1989), pp. 163–71.

74 V. Seidler (1997). *Man Enough: Embodying Masculinities* (London: Sage), p. 186; R. Connell (1995). *Masculinities* (Cambridge: Polity Press).

75 V. Seilder (1997).

76 J. Phillips (1996).

77 D. Sabo and F. Gordon (eds) (1995). *Men's Health and Illness: Gender, Power, and the Body* (Thousand Oaks: Sage), p. 16.

78 R. Connell (2000), p. 178.

79 J. Watson (2000), p. 2.

one
Masculinities and Globalisation

1 T. Carrigan, B. Connell and J. Lee, 'Toward a New Sociology of Masculinity', *Theory and Society*, 14 (5) (1985), pp. 551–604.

2 M.S. Kimmel (1987). 'Rethinking 'Masculinity': New Directions in Research', in M.S. Kimmel (ed.), *Changing Men: New Directions in Research on Men and Masculinity* (Newbury Park CA: Sage) pp. 9–24; R.W. Connell (1987). *Gender and Power* (Cambridge: Polity Press).

3 T. Carrigan *et al.* (1985); J. Hearn (1987). *The Gender of Oppression: Men, Masculinity and the Critique of Marxism* (Brighton: Wheatsheaf).

4 C. Cockburn (1983). *Brothers: Male Dominance and Technological Change*

(London: Pluto).

5 G.H. Herdt (1981). *Guardians of the Flutes: Idioms of Masculinity* (New York: McGraw-Hill).

6 R.W. Connell (1995). *Masculinities* (Cambridge: Polity Press); *Widersprueche* (1995) Special issue: 'Maennlichkeiten' vol. 56/57; L. Segal (1997). *Slow Motion: Changing Masculinities, Changing Men*, second edition (London: Virago).

7 J. Tosh (1991). 'Domesticity and Manliness in the Victorian Middle Class: the Family of Edward White Benson', in M. Roper and J. Tosh (eds), *Manful Assertions: Masculinities in Britain since 1800* (London: Routledge), pp. 44–73.

8 M.A. Messner (1992). *Power at Play: Sports and the Problem of Masculinity* (Boston: Beacon Press).

9 R.W. Connell, 'A Very Straight Gay: Masculinity, Homosexual Experience, and the Dynamics of Gender', *American Sociological Review* 57(6) (1992), pp. 735–751.

10 A.M. Klein (1993). *Little Big Men: Bodybuilding Subculture and Gender Construction* (Albany NY: State University of New York Press).

11 R. Morrell, 'Boys, Gangs and the Making of Masculinity in the White Secondary Schools of Natal, 1880–1930', *Masculinities* 2(2) (1994), pp. 56–82.

12 B. McElhinny (1994). 'An Economy of Effect: Objectivity, Masculinity and the Gendering of Police Work', in A. Cornwall and N. Lindisfarne (eds), *Dislocating Masculinity: Comparative Ethnographies* (London: Routledge), pp. 159–171.

13 S. Tomsen, 'A Top Night: Social Protest, Masculinity and the Culture of Drinking Violence', *British Journal of Criminology* 37 (1) (1997), pp. 90–103.

14 J.W. Messerschmidt (1997). *Crime as Structured Action: Gender, Race, Class, and Crime in the Making* (Thousand Oaks: Sage).

15 G.H. Herdt (ed.) (1984). *Ritualized Homosexuality in Melanesia* (Berkeley: University of California Press).

16 P. Hondagneu-Sotelo and M. A. Messner (1994). 'Gender Displays and Men's Power: The "New Man" and the Mexican Immigrant Man', in H. Brod and M. Kaufman (eds), *Theorizing Masculinities* (Thousand Oaks, CA: Sage), pp. 200–218.

17 D.E. Foley (1990). *Learning Capitalist Culture: Deep in the Heart of Tejas* (Philadelphia, University of Pennsylvania Press).

18 J.M. Messerschmidt (1997).

19 F.J. Barrett, 'The Organizational Construction of Hegemonic Masculinity: the Case of the U.S. Navy', *Gender, Work and Organization* 3(3) (1996), pp. 129–142.

20 J. McKay and D. Huber, 'Anchoring Media Images of Technology and Sport', *Women's Studies International Forum* 15(2) (1992), pp. 205–218.

21 R.W. Connell, 'The State, Gender and Sexual Politics: Theory and Appraisal', *Theory and Society* 19 (1990), pp. 507–544.

22 C. Cockburn (1983).

23 M. Donaldson (1991). *Time of Our Lives: Labour and Love in the Working Class* (Sydney: Allen and Unwin).

24 D. Whitson (1990). 'Sport in the Social Construction of Masculinity', in M.A. Messner and D.F. Sabo (eds), *Sport, Men, and the Gender Order: Critical Feminist Perspectives* (Champaign IL: Human Kinetics Books), pp. 19–29; M.A. Messner (1992).

25 R.W. Connell, 'Teaching the Boys: New Research on Masculinity, and Gender Strategies for Schools', *Teachers College Record* 98(2) (1996), pp. 206–235.

26 F.J. Barrett (1996).

27 N. Theberge, 'Reflections on the Body in the Sociology of Sport', *Quest* 43 (1991), pp. 123–134.

28 M. Donaldson (1991).

29 A. Bolin (1988). *In Search of Eve: Transsexual Rites of Passage* (Massachusetts: Bergin and Garvey).

30 M.A. Messner (1992).

31 J.C. Walker (1988). *Louts and Legends: Male Youth Culture in an Inner-City School* (Sydney: Allen and Unwin); B. Thorne (1993). *Gender Play: Girls and Boys in School* (New Brunswick: Rutgers University Press).

32 A.M. Klein (1993).

33 See N. Chodorow (1994). *Femininities, Masculinities, Sexualities: Freud and Beyond* (Lexington: University Press of Kentucky); K. Lewes (1988). *The Psychoanalytic Theory of Male Homosexuality* (New York: Simon and Schuster).

34 R.W. Connell (1995).

35 C. Heward (1988). *Making a Man of Him: Parents and their Sons' Education at an English Public School 1929–1950* (London: Routledge).

36 M. Roper (1991). 'Yesterday's Model: Product Fetishism and the British Company Man, 1945–85', in M. Roper and J. Tosh (eds), *Manful Assertions: Masculinities in Britain since 1800* (London: Routledge), pp. 190–211.

37 M. Schwalbe (1996). *Unlocking the Iron Cage: The Men's Movement, Gender Politics, and the American Culture* (New York: Oxford University Press).

38 M. Messner (1997). *The Politics of Masculinities: Men in Movements* (Thousand Oaks: Sage).

39 J. Phillips (1987). *A Man's Country? The Image of the Pakeha Male, A History* (Auckland: Penguin).

40 M.S. Kimmel (1996). *Manhood in America: A Cultural History* (New York: Free Press).

41 R.W. Connell (1990). 'An Iron Man: The Body and Some Contradictions of Hegemonic Masculinity', in M.A. Messner and D.F. Sabo (eds), *Sport, Men and the Gender Order: Critical Feminist Perspectives* (Champaign IL: Human Kinetics Books), pp. 83–95.

42 C. Enloe (1990). *Bananas, Beaches and Bases: Making Feminist Sense of International Politics* (Berkeley: University of California Press).

43 P. Hirst, and G. Thompson (1996). *Globalization in Question: The International Economy and the Possibilities of Governance* (Cambridge: Polity Press).

44 I. Wallerstein (1974*). The Modern World-System: Capitalist Agriculture and the Origins of the European World-Economy in the Sixteenth Century* (New York: Academic Press).

45 A. Fuentes and B. Ehrenreich (1983). *Women in the Global Factory* (Boston: South End Press).

46 R.W. Connell (1987); S. Walby (1990). *Theorizing Patriarchy* (Oxford: Blackwell).

47 M. Mies (1986). *Patriarchy and Accumulation on a World Scale: Women in the International Division of Labour* (London: Zed).

48 T.D. Moodie (1994). *Going for Gold: Men, Mines, and Migration* (Johannesburg: Witwatersrand University Press).

49 O.G. Holter (1997). *Gender, Patriarchy and Capitalism: A Social Forms Analysis* (PhD diss., Faculty of Social Science, University of Oslo).

50 D. Kandiyoti (1994). 'The Paradoxes of Masculinity: Some Thoughts on Segregated Societies', in A. Cornwall and N. Lindisfarne (eds), *Dislocating Masculinity: Comparative Ethnographies* (London: Routledge), pp. 197–213.

51 B. Hinsch (1990). *Passions of the Cut Sleeve: The Male Homosexual Tradition in China* (Berkeley: University of California Press).

52 D. Altman, 'Rupture or Continuity? The Internationalisation of Gay Identities', *Social Text* 48(3) (1996), pp. 77–94.

53 A. Simpson (1993). *Xuxa: The Mega-marketing of Gender, Race and Modernity* (Philadelphia: Temple University Press).

54 M. Jolly (1997). 'From Point Venus to Bali Ha'i: Eroticism and Exoticism in Representations of the Pacific', in L. Manderson and M. Jolly (eds), *Sites of Desire, Economies of Pleasure: Sexualities in Asia and the Pacific* (Chicago: University of Chicago Press), pp. 99–122.

55 R.W. Connell (1995).

56 U. Klein (1997). 'Our Best Boys: The Making of Masculinity in Israeli Society'. Paper to UNESCO expert group meeting on *Male Roles and Masculinities in the Perspectives of a Culture of Peace, Oslo*; G. Tillner (1997). 'Masculinity and Xenophobia'. Paper to UNESCO meeting on *Male Roles and Masculinities in the Perspective of a Culture of Peace, Oslo*.

57 S. Poynting, G. Noble and P. Tabar (1997). '"Intersections" of Masculinity and Ethnicity: A Study of Male Lebanese Immigrant Youth in Western Sydney'. Paper to Conference 'Masculinities: Renegotiating Genders' (University of Wollongong, June 1997).

58 R.W. Connell (1995).

59 M. Featherstone (1995). *Undoing Culture: Globalization, Postmodernism and Identity* (London: Sage).

60 W. Hollway (1994). 'Separation, Integration and Difference: Contradictions in a Gender Regime', in H.L. Radtke and H. Stam (eds), *Power/Gender: Social Relations in Theory and Practice* (London: Sage), pp. 247–269.

61 For example, D. Taylor (1985). 'Women: An Analysis', in *Women: A World Report* (London: Methuen), pp. 1–98.

62 U. Bitterli (1989). *Cultures in Conflict: Encounters Between European and Non-European Cultures, 1492–1800* (Stanford CA: Stanford University Press).

63 P.J. Cain and A.G. Hopkins (1993). *British Imperialism: Innovation and Expansion, 1688–1914* (New York: Longman).

64 J. Phillips (1987).

65 R. Morrell (1994).

66 U. Bitterli (1989).

67 T.D. Moodie (1994).

68 W.L. Williams (1986). *The Spirit and the Flesh: Sexual Diversity in American Indian Culture* (Boston: Beacon Press).

69 R. Morrell (ed.) (1996). *Political Economy and Identities in KwaZulu-Natal: Historical and Social Perspectives* (Durban: Indicator Press).

70 R.H. MacDonald (1994). *The Language of Empire: Myths and Metaphors of Popular Imperialism, 1880–1918* (Manchester: Manchester University Press).

71 C. Shire (1994). 'Men Don't Go to the Moon: Language, Space and Masculinities in Zimbabwe', in A. Cornwall and N. Lindisfarne (eds), *Dislocating Masculinity* (London: Routledge), pp.147–158.

72 M. Sinha (1995). *Colonial Masculinity: The 'Manly Englishman' and the 'Effeminate Bengali' in the late Nineteenth Century* (Manchester: Manchester University Press).

73 R. Kipling (1987). *Kim* (London: Penguin, [1st pub. 1901]).

74 C. Bulbeck (1992). *Australian Women in Papua New Guinea: Colonial Passages 1920–1960* (Cambridge, UK: Cambridge University Press).

75 G. Dawson (1991). 'The Blond Bedouin: Lawrence of Arabia, Imperial Adventure and the Imagining of English-British Masculinity', in M. Roper and J. Tosh (eds), *Manful Assertions: Masculinities in Britain since 1800* (London: Routledge), pp. 113–144.

76 E.H. Kinmonth (1981). *The Self-Made Man in Meiji Japanese Thought: From Samurai to Salary Man* (Berkeley: University of California Press).

77 M.S. Kimmel and T.E. Mosmiller (eds) (1992). *Against the Tide: Pro-Feminist Men in the United States, 1776–1990, A Documentary History* (Boston: Beacon Press).

78 G. Tillner (1997).

79 T. Xaba, 'Masculinity in a Transitional Society: The Rise and Fall of the 'Young Lions''. Paper presented at conference on Masculinities (Southern Africa: University of Natal-Durban, June 1997).

80 For example, M. Donaldson, 'Growing Up Very Rich: The Masculinity of the Hegemonic'. Paper to conference on *Masculinities: Renegotiating Genders* (University of Wollongong, 20 June 1997).

81 J.P. Gee, G. Hull and C. Lankshear (1996). *The New Work Order: Behind the Language of the New Capitalism* (Sydney: Allen and Unwin).

82 M. Messner (1997).

83 J.W. Gibson (1994). *Warrior Dreams: Paramilitary Culture in Post-Vietnam America* (New York: Hill and Wang).

84 D. Altman (1997).

85 J. Cohen, 'NOMAS: Challenging Male Supremacy', *Changing Men*, 10th Anniversary Issue (Winter/Spring) (1991), pp. 45–46.

86 V.J. Seidler (1991). *Achilles Heel Reader: Men, Sexual Politics and Socialism* (London: Routledge).

87 M. Kaufman (1997). 'Working with Men and Boys to Challenge Sexism and End Men's Violence'. Paper to UNESCO expert group meeting on *Male Roles and Masculinities in the Perspective of a Culture of Peace*, Oslo.

88 S. Metz-Goeckel and U. Mueller (1986). *Der Mann: Die Brigitte-Studie* [The male] (Beltz: Weinheim & Basel); C. Hagemann-White and M.S. Rerrich (eds) (1988). *FrauenMaennerBilder* [Women, Imaging, Men] (Bielefeld: AJZ-Verlag).

89 H. Kindler (1993). *Maske(r)ade: Jungen- und Maennerarbeit fuer die Praxis* (Schwaebisch Gmuend und Tuebingen: Neuling).

90 W. Hollstein (1992). *Machen Sie Platz mein Herr! Teilen statt Herrschen* [Sharing instead of dominating] (Hamburg: Rowohlt).

91 Widersprueche (1995); BauSteineMaenner (ed.) (1996). *Kritische Maennerforschung* (Berlin: Argument).

92 Gender Equality Ombudsman (1997). *The Father's Quota* [Information sheet on parental leave entitlements.] Oslo.

93 Ito Kimio (1993). *Otokorashisa-no-yukue* [Directions for Masculinities] (Tokyo: Shinyo-sha); Nakamura Akira (1994). *Watashi-no Danseigaku* [My Men's Studies] (Tokyo: Kindaibugei-sha).

94 United Nations Educational, Scientific and Cultural Organization (UNESCO) (1997). *Male Roles and Masculinities in the Perspective of a Culture of Peace: Report of Expert Group Meeting,* Oslo, Norway, 24–28 September 1997 (Paris: Women and a Culture of Peace Programme, Culture of Peace Unit, UNESCO).

95 A. Cornwall, and N. Lindisfarne (eds) (1994). *Dislocating Masculinity: Comparative Ethnographies* (London: Routledge); UNESCO (1997).

two

A Late Twentieth-Century Auckland Perspective on Samoan Masculinities

1 B. Shore (1981). 'Sexuality and Gender in Samoa', in S. Ortner and H. Whitehead (eds), *Sexual Meanings: the Cultural Construction of Gender and Sexuality* (Cambridge: Cambridge University Press), pp. 192–215.

2 For example, P. Schoeffel (1979). *Daughters of Sina: a Study of Gender, Status and Power in Western Samoa.* Unpublished PhD thesis in Anthropology, Australian National University, Canberra.

3 G. Rubin (1975). 'The Traffic in Women', in R. Reiter (ed.), *Toward an Anthropology of Women* (New York: Monthly Review), pp. 159.

4 Ibid. (1994), p. 90.

5 For example, P. Jackson (1986). 'Man<>Kathoey<>Gay', in L. Manderson and M. Jolly (eds), *Sites of Desire* (Chicago: Chicago University Press), pp. 166–190; H. Moore (1999). 'Whatever Happened to Women and Men? Gender and other Crises in Anthropology', in H.L. Moore (ed.), *Anthropological Theory Today* (Cambridge: Polity Press), pp. 151–171.

6 P. Schoeffel (1979), p. 230; S. Ortner (1981). 'Gender and Sexuality in Hierarchical Societies: the Case of Polynesia', in S. Ortner and H. Whitehead (eds), *Sexual Meanings: the Cultural Construction of Gender and Sexuality* (Cambridge: Cambridge University Press), p. 394; B. Shore (1981), p. 200ff.

7 P. Schoeffel (1979).

8 Ibid. (1979), p. 297.

9 T. Sua'ali'a (2001). 'Samoans and Gender: Some Reflections on Male, Female and Fa'afafine Gender Identities', in C. Macpherson, P. Spoonley and M. Anae (eds), *Tangata o te Moana Nui: The Evolving Identities of Pacific Peoples in Aotearoa/New Zealand* (Palmerston North: Dunmore).

10 B. Shore (1981).

11 J. Park (ed.) (1991). *Ladies a Plate: Change and Continuity in the Lives of New Zealand Women* (Auckland: Auckland University Press), p. 28.

12 M. Anae *et al.* (2000).

13 V. Krishnan, P. Schoeffel and J. Warren (1994). *The Challenge of Change: Pacific Island Communities in New Zealand 1986–1993.* (Wellington, New Zealand: Institute for Social Research and Development), p. 17.

14 New Zealand Ministry of Pacific Island Affairs (1999). *Social Economic Status of Pacific People Report* (Wellington, Ministry of Pacific Island Affairs), p. 14.

15 See M. Anae (1998).

16 New Zealand Ministry of Pacific Island Affairs (1999), p. 5.

17 V. Krishnan *et al.* (1994).

18 Ibid (1994), p. 30.

19 Statistics New Zealand (1998). *Census 1996: Pacific Islands People* (Wellington: Statistics New Zealand); C. Tukuitonga, 'Pacific Peoples in New Zealand, *Pacific Health Dialog* 4(2) (1997), pp. 4–5.

20 See Anae *et al.* (2000), p. 253ff for details.

21 P. Schoeffel (1979).

22 M. Mead (1943). *Coming of Age in Samoa* (London: Penguin Books), p. 29; P. Schoeffel (1979), p. 184; S. Tcherkézoff (2001). *Le Mythe Occidental de la Sexualité Polynésienne: 1928–1999; Margaret Mead, Derek Freeman et Samoa* (Paris: Presses Universitaires de France), p. 45.

23 R.W. Connell (1995) *Masculinities* (St Leonards: Allen and Unwin), p. 46.

three

Living the Contradictions: A Foucauldian Examination of my Youthful Rugby Experiences

1 S. Coney, *Kiwi Just Another Brand Name* (*New Zealand Herald*, 5 September, 1999), p. C4, C5.

2 S. Zavos (1988). 'In Praise of Rugby', in M. King (ed.), *One of the Boys? Changing Views of Masculinity in New Zealand* (Auckland: Heinemann), p. 119.

3 E. Dunning and K. Sheard (1979). *Barbarians, Gentlemen and Players: A Sociological Study of the Development of Rugby Football* (Oxford: Martin Robertson).

4 C. Laidlaw (1999). 'Sport and National Identity: Race Relations, Business, Professionalism', in B. Patterson (ed.), *Sport, Society & Culture in New Zealand* (Palmerston North: The Dunmore Press), pp. 11–18.

5 T. Richards (1999). 'New Zealanders' Attitudes to Sport as Illustrated by Debate over Rugby Contacts with South Africa', in B. Patterson (ed.), *Sport, Society & Culture in New Zealand* (Palmerston North: Dunmore), pp. 39–48.

6 S. Thompson (1988), 'Challenging the Hegemony: New Zealand's Women's Opposition to Rugby and the Reproduction of Capitalist Patriarch', *International Review for the Sociology of Sport* 23(2), pp. 205–223.

7 J. Ritchie and J. Ritchie (1993). *Violence in New Zealand* (Wellington: Daphne Brasell Associates).

8 Ibid (1993), p. 100.

9 J.R. Nauright (1996). 'Sustaining Masculine Hegemony: Rugby and the Nostalgia of Masculinity', in J. Nauright and T. Chandler (eds), *Making Men: Rugby and Masculine Identity* (London: Frank Cass & Co), pp. 227–244.

10 R.C. McConnell (1998). *Inside the All Blacks* (Auckland: HarperCollins), p. 11.

11 R.W. Connell (1995). *Masculinities* (St Leonards: Allen and Unwin); M. A. Messner, 'Men Studying Masculinity: Some Epistemological Issues in Sport Sociology', *Sociology of Sport Journal* 7 (1990), pp. 136–153; A.C. Sparkes and B. Smith (1999). 'Disrupted Selves and Narrative Reconstructions', in A.C. Sparkes and M. Silvennolnen (eds), *Talking Bodies* (Jyvaskyla: SoPhi), pp. 76–91.

12 M.A. Messner (1994). 'Sports and Male Domination: The Female Athlete as Contested Ideological Terrain', in S. Birrell and C. Cole (eds), *Women, Sport, and Culture* (Champaign, IL: Human Kinetics), p. 67.

13 A. Gray (1983). *The Jones Men: 100 New Zealand Men Talk About their Lives* (Wellington: Reed), p. 29.

14 J. Phillips (1996). 'The Hard Man: Rugby and the Formation of Male Identity in New Zealand', in J. Nauright and T. Chandler (eds), *Making Men: Rugby and Masculine Identity* (London: Frank Cass), pp. 70–90.

15 Ibid.

16 Ibid.

17 L. Star (1999a). "'Blacks are Back': Ethnicity, Male Bodies, Exhibitionary Order', in R. Law, H. Campbell and J. Dolan (eds), *Masculinities in Aotearoa/New Zealand* (Palmerston North: Dunmore Press), p. 231.

18 J. Park . 'The Worst Hassle Is You Can't Play Rugby': Haemophilia and Masculinity in New Zealand', *Current Anthropology* 41(3) (2000), p. 446.

19 Ibid. p. 445.

20 J. Coakley (1994). *Sport in Society: Issues and Controversies* (St Louis: Mosby), p. 172.

21 N. Trujillo. 'Machines, Missiles, and Men: Images of the Male Body on ABC's Monday Night Football', *Sociology of Sport Journal,* (1995), 12 pp. 403–423.

22 L. Star. 'Televised Rugby and Male Violence', *New Zealand Journal of Media Studies* 1(1) (1994), pp. 33–45.

23 Accident Rehabilitation and Compensation Insurance Corporation (1998). *ACC Entitlement Claims Statistics for Rugby Union Injuries: October* (ACC Scheme Forecasting and Reporting Unit).

24 Ibid.

25 J. Ritchie (1981). 'Boys will be Boys: New Zealanders' Approval of Violence'. Paper presented at *Proceedings: Women's Studies Association Conference* (Wellington, 1981), pp. 129–140; L. Star (1994); S. Thompson (1988); M.J. Trevelyan and S. Jackson (1999). 'Clash of the Codes: A Comparative Analysis of Media Representation of Violence in Rugby Union and Rugby League', in J. Nauright (ed.), *Sport, Power and Society in New Zealand: Historical and Contemporary Perspectives* (ASSH Studies in Sport History no. 11), pp. 113–138.

26 J. Kenway and L. Fitzclarence, 'Masculinity, Violence and Schooling: Challenging "Poisonous Pedagogies"', *Gender and Education* 9 (1) (1997), pp. 117–133.

27 J. Ritchie and J. Ritchie (1993). p. vii.

28 P. Adams (1997). 'Men', in P. Ellis (ed.), *Mental Health in New Zealand From a Public Health Perspective* (Wellington: Public Health Group, Ministry of Health), pp. 213–242.

29 J. Kenway and L. Fitzclarence (1997), p. 122.

30 H.L. II Nixon. 'Gender, Sport, and Aggressive Behaviour Outside Sport', *Journal of Sport and Social Issues*, 21(4) (1997), pp. 379–391.

31 T. W. Crosset, J.R. Benedict and M.A. McDonald. 'Male Student-Athletes Reported for Sexual Assault: A Survey of Campus Police Departments and Judicial Affairs Offices', *Journal of Sport and Social Issues* 19 (1995), pp. 126–140.

32 J. Ritchie (1981).

33 J-F. Lyotard (1984) *The Postmodern Condition: A Report on Knowledge* (Manchester: Manchester University Press).

34 J. Phillips (1996).

35 R. Lynch. 'The Cultural Repositioning of Rugby League and its Men', *ANZALS Leisure Research Series* Vol 1 (1993), pp. 105–119; H. Yeates, 'The League of Men: Masculinity, the Media and Rugby League', *Media Information Australia* 75 (1995), pp. 35–45.

36 G. Whannel. 'Sport Stars, Narrativization and Masculinities', *Leisure Studies* 18 (1999), p. 252.

37 Ibid, p. 253.

38 For example: S.L. Bartky (1988). 'Foucault, Femininity, and the Modernization of Patriarchal Power', in I. Diamond and L. Quinby (eds), *Feminism and Foucault: Reflections on Resistance* (Boston: Northeastern University Press), pp. 61–86; S. Bordo (1988). 'Anorexia Nervosa: Psychopathology as the Crystallization of Culture', in I. Diamond and L. Quinby (eds), *Feminism and Foucault: Reflections on Resistance* (Boston: Northeastern University Press), pp. 87–117; J. Butler (1990). *Gender Trouble: Feminism and the Subversion of Identity* (New York: Routledge); C.L. Cole (1994). 'Resisting the Canon: Feminist Cultural Studies, Sport, and Technologies of the Body', in S. Birrell and C. Cole (eds), *Women, Sport, and Culture* (Champaign, IL: Human Kinetics), pp. 5–29; I. Diamond and L. Quinby (1988). 'Introduction', in I. Diamond and L. Quinby (eds), *Feminism and Foucault: Reflections on Resistance* (Boston, MA: Northeastern University Press), pp. ix–xx; J. Sawicki (1988). 'Identity Politics and Sexual Freedom: Foucault and Feminism', in I. Diamond and L. Quinby (eds), *Feminism and Foucault: Reflections on Resistance* (Boston, MA: Northeastern University Press), pp. 177–191; J. Sawicki (1991). *Disciplining Foucault: Feminism, Power, and the Body* (New York, NY: Routledge); E. Sedgwick (1995). 'Gosh, Boy George, You must be Awfully Secure in your Masculinity', in M. Berger, B. Wallis and S. Watson (eds), *Constructing Masculinity* (New York: Routledge), pp. 11–20; C. Weedon (1987). *Feminist Practice and Poststructuralist Theory* (Oxford: Blackwell).

39 L. Star (1999). 'New Masculinities Theory: Poststructuralism and Beyond', in R. Law, H. Campbell and J. Dolan (eds), *Masculinities in Aotearoa/New Zealand* (Palmerston North: Dunmore Press), pp. 36–45.

40 M. Foucault (1988). 'Technologies of the Self', in L.H. Martin, H. Gutman, and P.H. Hutton (eds), *Technologies of the Self: A Seminar with Michel Foucault* (Amherst: University of Massachusetts Press), pp. 17–18.

41 M. Foucault (1972). *The Archaeology of Knowledge* (trans. by A.M. Sheridan) (London: Routledge, original work published 1969), p. 49.

42 M. Foucault (1978). *The History of Sexuality, Volume 1: An Introduction* (trans. R. Hurley) (New York, NY: Random House, original work published 1976), p. 100.

43 M. Foucault (1978).

44 M. Foucault (1988), p. 10.

45 V. Burr (1995). *An Introduction to Social Constructionism* (London: Routledge), p. 90.

46 M. Foucault (1978), p. 100.

47 Ibid.

48 Ibid, p. 94.

49 J. Sawicki (1991), p. 23.

50 R.W. Connell (1995).

51 T. Carrigan, R. Connell and J. Lee (1987) 'Hard and Heavy: Toward a New Sociology of Masculinity', in M. Kaufman (ed.), *Beyond Patriarchy: Essays by Men on Pleasure, Power and Change* (Toronto: Oxford University), pp. 179.

52 L. Star (1999), 'New Masculinities Theory: Poststructuralism and Beyond', in R. Law, H. Campbell and J. Dolan (eds), *Masculinities in Aotearoa/New Zealand* (Palmerston North: Dunmore Press), p. 40.

53 M. Donaldson, 'What is Hegemonic Masculinity?', *Theory and Society* 22 (5) (1993), pp. 643–657; N. Edley and M. Wetherell, 'Negotiating Hegemonic Masculinity: Imaginary Positions and Psycho-Discursive Practices', *Discourse and Society* 8 (2) (1999), pp. 203–217; T. Miller, 'Commodifying the Male Body, Problematising 'Hegemonic Masculinity?', *Journal of Sport and Social Issues* 22 (4) (1998), pp. 431–447; L. Star (1999).

54 T. Miller (1998), p. 433.

55 M. Foucault (1978), p. 101.

56 M. Foucault (1973). *The Birth of the Clinic: An Archaeology of Medical Perception* (trans. A. M. Sheridan Smith) (New York, NY: Pantheon, original work published 1963).

57 P. Rabinow (1984). 'Space, Knowledge and Power (An Interview with Michel Foucault)', in P. Rabinow (ed.), *The Foucault Reader* (New York: Pantheon Books), p. 8.

58 B. Smart (1985). *Michel Foucault* (Chichester: Ellis Horword Limited).

59 D. Knights. 'Changing Spaces: The Disruptive Impact of a New Epistemological Allocation for the Study of Management', *Academy of Management Review* 17 (3) (1992), p. 518.

60 M. Foucault (1988), p. 18.

61 M. Foucault (1977). *Discipline and Punish: The Birth of the Prison* (trans. by A. M. Sheridan) (New York: Pantheon Books, original work published 1975), p. 137.

62 B. Smart (1985), p. 85.

63 P. Rabinow (1984); B. Smart (1985).

64 Cited in R. Fornet-Betancourt, H. Becker and A. Gomez-Muller (1994). 'The Ethic of Care for the Self as a Practice of Freedom: An Interview with Michel Foucault', in J. Bernauer and D. Rasmussen (eds), *The Final Foucault* (Cambridge, MA: The MIT Press), p. 2.

65 M. Foucault in Fornet-Betancourt *et al.* (1994), p. 11.

66 A. Sparkes (1997). 'Reflections on the Socially Constructed Self', in K.R. Fox (ed.), *The Physical Self: From Motivation to Well-Being* (Champaign, IL: Human Kinetics), pp. 83–110.

67 S. Hall (1992). 'The Question of Cultural Identity', in S. Hall, D. Hell, and T. McGrew (eds), *Modernity and its Futures* (Cambridge: Polity), pp. 374–425.

68 N. Edley and M. Wetherell (1997). 'Jockeying for Position: The Construction of Masculine Identities', *Discourse & Society* 8 (2) (1997), pp. 203–217; C.A. Hasbrook and O. Harris, 'Wrestling with Gender: Physicalities and Masculinities Among Inner-City First and Second Graders', *Men and Masculinities* 1 (3) (1999), pp. 302–318; E. Jordan, 'Fighting Boys and Fantasy Play: The Construction of Masculinity in the Early Years of School', *Gender and Education* 7(1) (1995), pp. 69–86; A. Parker, 'The Construction of Masculinity within Boys' Physical Education', *Gender and Education* 8 (2) (1996), pp. 141–157; C. Skelton, 'Learning to be 'Tough': The Fostering of Maleness in One Primary School', *Gender and Education* 8 (2) (1996), pp. 185–197; J. Swain, 'The Money's Good, the Fame's Good, the Girls are Good': The Role of Playground Football in the Construction of Young Boys' Masculinity in a Junior School', *British Journal Of Sociology of Education* 21 (1) (2000), pp. 95–109.

69 C. Skelton (2000). 'A Passion for Football': Dominant Masculinities and Primary Schooling', *Sport, Education and Society* 5 (1), p. 5.

70 N. Edley and M. Wetherell (1997), p. 207.

71 M. Foucault (1977). p. 25.

72 J. Butler (1990), p. 33.

73 L. Star (1994).

74 D. Rowe (1995). 'Big Defence: Sport and Hegemonic Masculinity', in A. Tomlinson (ed.), *Gender, Sport and Leisure: Continuities and Challenges* (University of Brighton: Chelsea School Research Centre), pp. 123–133.

75 G. Fougere (1989). 'Sport, Culture, and Identity: The Case of Rugby Football', in D. Novitz and B. Willmont (eds), *Culture and Identity in New Zealand* (Wellington: GP Books), p. 111.

four

Managing the Margins: Gay-Disabled Masculinity

1 B. Cruikshank (1996). 'Revolutions Within Self-Government and Self-Esteem', in A. Barry, T. Osborne and N. Rose (eds), *Foucault and Political Reason: Liberalism, Neo-liberalism and Rationalities of Government* (London: UCL Press).

2 E. Said (1979). *Orientalism* (New York: Vintage Books).

3 L. Nencel (1996). 'Pancharacas, Putas and Chicas de su Casa: Labelling, Femininity and Men's Sexual Selves in Lima, Peru', in M. Melhuus and K.A. Stolen (eds), *Machos, Mistresses, Madonnas* (London and New York: Verso).

4 T. Miller (1993). *The Well-Tempered Self: Citizenship, Culture, and the Postmodern Subject* (Baltimore: John Hopkins University Press).

5 C. Mouffe (1988). 'Sexuality, Regulation and Contestation', in Gay Left Collective (ed), *Homosexuality: Power and Politics* (London: Allison and Busby).

6 N. Duncan (1996). 'Introduction: (Re)placings', in N. Duncan (ed), *Bodyspace: Destabilising Geographies of Gender and Sexuality* (London and New York: Routledge).

7 L. McDowell (1996). 'Spatializing Feminism: Geographic Perspectives', in N. Duncan (ed.), *Bodyspace: Destabilising Geographies of Gender and Sexuality* (London and New York: Routledge).

8 E.P. Archetti (1996). 'Playing Styles and Masculine Virtues in Argentine Football', in M. Melhuss and K.A. Stolen (eds), *Machos, Mistresses, Madonnas* (London and New York: Verso).

9 N.J. Chowdorow (1994). *Femininities, Masculinities, Sexualities* (Kentucky: University of Kentucky Press), p. 91.

10 N. Rose (1996). 'Governing 'Advanced' Liberal Democracies', in A. Barry, T. Osborne and N. Rose (eds), *Foucault and Political Reason: Liberalism, Neo-Liberalism and Rationalities of Government* (London: UCL Press).

11 T. Miller (1993).

12 A. Barry, T. Osborne and N. Rose (eds) (1996). *Foucault and Political Reason: Liberalism, Neo-Liberalism and Rationalities of Government* (London: UCL Press), p. 1.

13 G. Burchell (1991). 'Peculiar Interests: Civil Society and Governing 'The System of Natural Liberty', in G. Burchell, G. Gordon and P. Miller (eds), *The Foucault Effect: Studies in Governmentality* (Chicago: University of Chicago Press), p. 122.

14 N. Rose in A. Barry *et al.* (1996), p. 59.

15 J. Minson (1993). *Questions of Conduct: Sexual Harassment, Citizenship and*

Government (London: Macmillan).

16 M. Foucault (1979). *The History of Sexuality, Volume 1: An Introduction* (trans. R. Hurley) (London: Allen Lane).

17 W.G. Tierney (1997). *Academic Outlaws: Queer Theory and Cultural Studies in the Academy* (Thousand Oaks, CA: Sage); J.E. Toews (1994). 'Foucault and the Foucauldian Subject: Archaeology, Genealogy and the Historicisation of Psychoanalysis', in J. Goldstein (ed.), *Foucault and the Writing of History* (Oxford, UK and Cambridge, Mass: Blackwell).

18 A. Giddens (1991). *Modernity and Self Identity: Self and Society in the Late Modern Age* (Cambridge: Polity Press).

19 A. McHoul and W. Grace (1998). *A Foucault Primer: Discourse, Power and the Subject* (Dunedin: University of Otago Press).

20 C. Boggs (1986). *Social Movements and Political Power* (Philadelphia: Temple University Press), p. 4.

21 R.W. Connell (1987). *Gender and Power: Society, the Person and Sexual Politics* (Cambridge: Polity Press), p. 25.

22 N. Rose in A. Barry *et al.* (1996), p. 59.

five

'I DIDN'T HAVE TO GO TO A FINISHING SCHOOL TO LEARN HOW TO BE GAY': MAORI GAY MEN'S UNDERSTANDINGS OF CULTURAL AND SEXUAL IDENTITY

1 H.W. Williams (1992). *A Dictionary of the Maori Language* (Wellington: Government Printer).

2 J. Linnekin and L. Poyer (1990). 'Introduction', in J. Linnekin and L. Poyer (eds), *Cultural Identity and Ethnicity in the Pacific* (Honolulu: University of Hawaii Press).

3 R.C. Bleys (1995). *The Geography of Perversion* (Washington Square, NY: New York University Press).

4 T. Tafoya (1992). 'Native Gay and Lesbian Issues: The Two-Spirited', in B. Berzon (ed.), *Positively Gay. New Approaches to Gay and Lesbian Life* (Berkeley, CA: Celestial Arts Publishing).

5 S-E. Jacobs (1997). 'Is the 'North American Berdache' Merely a Phantom in the Imagination of Western Social Scientists?', in S-E. Jacobs, W. Thomas and S. Lang (eds), *Two-Spirit People. Native American Gender Identity, Sexuality and Spirituality* (Urbana and Chicago: University of Illinois Press).

6 R.C. Bleys (1995), p. 23.

7 E.W. Said (1978), *Orientalism. Western Conceptions of the Orient* (London: Penguin Books), p. 332.

8 L. Kahaleole Chang Hall and K.J. Kehaulani (1996), 'Same-Sex Sexuality in Pacific Literature', in R. Leong (eds), *Asian American Sexualities. Dimensions of Gay and Lesbian Experience* (New York: Routledge), p. 114.

9 N. Te Awekotuku (1991). *Mana Wahine: Selected Writings on Maori Women's Art, Culture and Politics* (Auckland: New Women's Press), p. 38.

10 Ibid, p. 32.

11 T. Karetu (1995). *Te Tau o te Reo Maori: the Influence of the Maori Language* (Te Puni Kokiri, Wellington).

12 T. Herewini, personal communication.

13 T. Herewini and R.H. Sheridan (1994). *A Report on the Health Needs of Maori*

Gay Men (Wellington: Public Health Commission), p. 4.

14 E-S. Gutierrez (1992). 'Latino Issues: Gay and Lesbian Latinos Claiming La Raza', in B. Berzon (ed.), *Positively Gay. New Approaches to Gay and Lesbian Life* (Berkeley, CA: Celestial Arts), p. 241.

15 L.D. Icard (1996). 'Assessing the Psychosocial Well-Being of African American Gays: A Multidimensional Perspective', in J.F. Longres (ed.), *Men of Colour. A Context for Service to Homosexually Active Men* (Binghamton, NY: Harrington Park Press), p. 149.

16 C.A. Aspin, C.A. Reid, H. Worth, P. Saxton, T. Hughes, E. Robinson and R. Segedin (1998). *Male Call/Waea Mai, Tane Ma. Report Three: Mäori Men Who Have Sex with Men* (Auckland: New Zealand AIDS Foundation).

17 T.S. Weinberg, 'On 'Doing' and 'Being' Gay: Sexual Behavior and Homosexual Male Self-identity', *Journal of Homosexuality* 4 (1978), pp. 143–157; J. Weeks (1991). *Against Nature: Essays on History, Sexuality and Identity* (London: Rivers Oram Press).

18 J. Weeks (1985). *Sexuality and its Discontents. Meanings, Myths and Modern Sexualities* (London: Routledge and Kegan Paul), p. 189.

19 M. McCarthy (1997). 'Raising a Maori Child Under a New Right State', in P. Te Whaiti, M. McCarthy, and A. Durie (eds), *Mai i Rangiatea* (Auckland: Auckland University Press with Bridget Williams Books).

six

The Man with Two Brains

1 J. Lacan (1977). *Ecrits: A Selection* (trans. A. Sheridan) (London: Routledge, original work pub. 1966).

2 See A. Potts. '"The Essence of the Hard On": Hegemonic Masculinity and the Cultural Construction of "Erectile Dysfunction"', *Men and Masculinities* 3 (1) (2000), pp. 85–103.

3 J. Derrida (1981). *Dissemination* (trans. B. Johnson) (Chicago: The University of Chicago Press), p. 103.

4 E. Grosz (1994). *Volatile Bodies: Toward a Corporeal Feminism* (St Leonards, NSW: Allen & Unwin), p. vii.

5 B. Wearing (1996). *Gender: The Pain and Pleasure of Difference* (Melbourne: Longman Australia), p. 68.

6 R. Braidotti (1994). *Nomadic Subjects: Embodiment and Sexual Difference in Contemporary Feminist Theory* (New York: Columbia University Press), p. 3.

7 E. Grosz (1994); see also J-F. Lyotard, (1993). *Libidinal Economy* (trans. I. H. Grant), (Bloomington: Indiana University Press, original work pub. 1974 by Les Editions De Minuit, Paris).

8 *Collins English Dictionary,* (1986) 2nd ed. (London: Collins), p. 989.

9 E. Grosz (1994).

10 Twenty women and seventeen men were involved in this study, participating in either individual interviews or same-sex group discussions facilitated by the author. All participants identified as Pakeha New Zealanders (i.e. non-Maori, of European descent). Ages ranged from twenty to forty-eight years. To ensure confidentiality, the names of participants have been changed. Italicised parts of transcripts indicate where the speaker has emphasised a word or phrase.

11 D. Massey (1996). 'Masculinity, Dualisms and High Technology', in N. Duncan (ed.), *BodySpace: Destabilizing Geographies of Gender and Sexuality* (London: Routledge), p. 121.

12 Ibid. (1996).

13 L. Irigaray (1993). *An Ethics of Sexual Difference* (trans. C. Burke and G.C. Gill) (Ithaca, New York: Cornell University Press, original work pub. 1984), p. 63.

14 M. Whitford (1991). *Luce Irigaray: Philosophy in the Feminine* (London: Routledge), p. 88.

15 L. Jordanova (1989). *Sexual Visions: Images of Gender in Science and Medicine Between the Eighteenth and Twentieth Centuries* (New York: Harvester Wheatsheaf).

16 For an analysis of male and female embodiment in environmental space, see Iris Marion Young (1990). *Throwing like a Girl and Other Essays in Feminist Philosophy and Social Theory* (Bloomington and Indianapolis: Indiana University Press).

17 C. Bernheimer (1995). 'A Question of Reference: Male Sexuality in Phallic Theory', in M. Cohen and C. Prendergast (eds), *Spectacles of Realism: Body, Gender, Genre* (Minneapolis: University of Minnesota Press), p. 326.

18 V. Kaplan (producer), and B. Gowers (director) (1986). *Robin Williams Live* [video]. (USA: Mr. Happy Productions Inc).

19 P. Lopate (1994). 'Portrait of my Body', in L. Goldstein (ed.), *The Male Body: Features, Destinies, Exposures* (Michigan: The University of Michigan Press), p. 211.

20 S. Frosh (1994). *Sexual Difference: Masculinity and Psychoanalysis* (London: Routledge), p. 104.

21 V. Seidler (1987). 'Reason, Desire, and Male Sexuality', in P. Caplan (ed.), *The Cultural Construction of Sexuality* (London: Tavistock Publications Limited).

22 Frosh (1994), p. 104.

23 My argument here contrasts with Victor Seidler's contention that the alliance between masculinity and reason has 'estranged "men" from their bodies' to such an extent that 'sexuality becomes primarily a mental experience for them'. See Seidler, (1987), p. 96.

24 H. Haste (1994). *The Sexual Metaphor* (Cambridge, Massachusetts: Harvard University Press).

25 E. Martin (1992). *The Woman in the Body: A Cultural Analysis of Reproduction* (Boston: Beacon Press).

26 M. FitzGerald (producer & director), and M. Coombes (director) (1994), *Sex, Guys and Videotape* [film documentary]. Australia: Australian Broadcasting Corporation.

27 See N. Gavey (1990). 'Feminist Poststructuralism and Discourse Analysis', *Psychology of Women Quarterly*, 13 (1989), pp. 459–475; *Rape and sexual coercion within heterosexual relationships: an intersection of psychological, feminist, and postmodern inquiries*, unpublished PhD thesis, University of Auckland; 'Technologies and Effects of Heterosexual Coercion', *Feminism & Psychology*, 2(3) (1992), pp. 325–351.

28 I would like to thank Philip Armstrong and Nicola Gavey for reading earlier drafts of this chapter and providing valuable comments. I would also like to thank those women and men who voluntarily participated in this study, and the New Zealand Health Research Council, the New Zealand Family Planning Association, the New Zealand Federation of University Women, and the Auckland University Graduate Research Committee for their financial support of this research.

seven

'Tits is Just an Accessory': Masculinity and Femininity in the Lives of Maori and Pacific Queens

1 V. Kirby (1997). *Telling Flesh: The Substance of the Corporeal* (New York: Routledge), p. 67.

2 J. Butler (1990). *Gender Trouble: Feminism and the Subversion of Identity* (London: Routledge), p. 25.

3 J. Butler (1993). *Bodies That Matter: On the Discursive Limits of 'Sex'* (New York: Routledge), p. 122.

4 Ibid., p. 230.

5 J. Butler (1990), p. 31.

6 G. Dowsett (1996). *Practicing Desire: Homosexual Sex in the Era of AIDS* (Stanford, California: Stanford University Press), p. 99.

7 N. Besnier (1994). 'Polynesian Gender Liminality Through Time and Space', in G. Herdt (ed.), *Third Sex, Third Gender: Beyond Sexual Dimorphism in Culture and History* (New York: Zone Books), p. 308.

8 Ibid., p. 304.

9 R.W. Connell (1995). *Masculinities: Knowledge, Power and Social Change* (Berkeley, California: California University Press), p. 77.

10 M. Foucault, *Ethics of Pleasure*, p. 380.

11 J. Butler (1993), p. 238.

12 Ibid., p. 235.

13 L. Pettiway (1996). *Honey, Honey, Miss Thang: Being Black, Gay and On the Streets* (Philadelphia: Temple University Press), p. xii.

14 G. Dowsett (1996). *Practicing Desire: Homosexual Sex in the Era of AIDS* (Stanford, California: Stanford University Press).

15 J. Butler (1993), pp. 126–7.

16 See J. Derrida (1991). 'At This Very Moment in This Work Here I Am', in R. Bernasconi and S. Critchley (eds), *Re-Reading Levinas* (trans. R. Berezdivin) (Bloomington and Indianapolis: Indiana University Press), pp. 11–49.

17 V. Kirby (1997), p. 137.

18 J. Derrida (1968). 'Difference', in *Margins of Philosophy* (trans. A. Bass) (Chicago: University of Chicago Press), pp. 3–27.

19 V. Kirby (1997), p. 95.

20 J. Butler (1993), p. 125.

21 J. Derrida (1992). 'The Law of Genre', in D. Attridge (ed.), *Acts of Literature* (New York: Routledge), pp. 224–5.

22 Ibid, p. 225.

23 V. Kirby (1995), p. 95.

24 Jacques Derrida (1991). 'Choreographies' in Peggy Konuf (ed.), *A Derrida Reader* (US: Harvester Wheatsheaf, p. 132.

25 V. Kirby (1995), p. 95.

26 Judith Butler (1990). *Gender Trouble: Feminism and the Subversion of Identity* (New York: Routledge), p. 54.

eight

'As Far as Sex Goes I Don't Really Think About My Body': Young Men's Corporeal Experiences of (Hetero)sexual Pleasure

1 K. Dutton (1995). *The Perfectible Body: The Western Ideal of Physical Development* (London: Cassell); D. Morgan (1993). 'You Too Can Have a Body Like Mine: Reflections on the Male Body and Masculinities', in S. Scott and D. Morgan (eds), *Body Matters: Essays on the Sociology of the Body* (London: Falmer); M. Featherstone, M. Hepworth and B. Turner (eds) (1991). *The Body: Social and Cultural Theory* (London: Sage); C. Waldby (1995). 'Destruction: Boundary Erotics and Reconfigurations of the Heterosexual Male Body' in E. Grosz and E. Probyn (eds), *Sexy Bodies: The Strange Carnalities of Feminism* (London: Routledge).

2 J. Stacey (1997). 'Feminist Theory: Capital F, Capital T', in V. Robinson and D. Richardson (eds), *Introducing Women's Studies* (London: MacMillian).

3 A. Parker (1996). 'Sporting Masculinities: Gender Relations and the Body', in M. Mac an Ghaill (ed.), *Understanding Masculinities* (Buckingham: Open University Press); B. Kidd (1987). 'Sports and Masculinity', in M. Kaufman (ed.), *Beyond Patriarchy* (New York: Oxford University Press); R. Majors (1990). 'Cool Pose: Black Masculinity and Sports', in M. Messener and D. Sabo (eds), *Sport, Men and the Gender Order* (Champaign: Human Kinetics); S. Gilroy, 'The EmBody-ment of Power: Gender and Physical Activity', *Leisure Studies* 8 (1989), pp. 163–71; T. Jefferson, 'Muscle, 'Hard Men' and 'Iron' Mike Tyson: Reflections on Desire, Anxiety and the Embodiment of Masculinity', *Body and Society* 4(1) (1998), pp. 77–98.

4 M. Corbett Robertson (1994). *Unruly Sites: Subjectivity and Masculine Enfleshment* Thesis submitted in partial fulfilment of Master of Arts in Psychology, University of Auckland; M. Lindner, R. Ryckman, J. Gold and W. Stone, 'Traditional vs. Nontraditional Women and Men's Perceptions of the Personalities and Physiques of Ideal Women and Men', *Sex Roles* 32(9/10) (1995), pp. 675–690.

5 Subjects were drawn from seven schools (n=342) and 18 Training Opportunity Programmes (n=173) designed to assist people to gain qualifications and skills for employment. The research sample was ethnically diverse with 57.4 per cent Pakeha (European), 16.3 per cent Maori, 16.3 per cent Pacific Islands, 9.1 Asian, 1 per cent other. Both single sex and mixed gender focus groups (17 in total) were undertaken with 5–10 subjects who were typically friends. 411 questionnaires exploring young people's conceptualisation of their sexual knowledge, subjectivities and heterosexual practices were completed. A couple activity was also undertaken, with six couples in a heterosexual relationship at the time of the research. This involved couples sorting cards with a series of phrases about their relationship into piles under three possible headings 'often happens or happened in our relationship', 'sometimes happens or happened in our relationship' and 'never happens in our relationship'. This was followed by an individual interview with each partner of the couple.

6 R. Connell (1995). *Masculinities* (Cambridge: Polity Press); V. Seidler (1997). *Man Enough: Embodying Masculinities* (London: Sage).

7 See for example, R. Weitz (ed.) (1998). *The Politics of Women's Bodies: Sexuality, Appearance and Behaviour* (New York: Oxford University Press); G. Weiss (1999).

Body Images: Embodiment as Intercorporeality (London: Routledge); J. Holland, C. Ramazanoglu, S. Sharpe and R. Thomson (1994). 'Power and Desire: The Embodiment of Female Sexuality', *Feminist Review* 46 (Spring) (1994); S. Williams (1996). 'The Vicissitudes of Embodiment Across the Chronic Illness Trajectory', *Body and Society* 2 (2) (1996); T. Jefferson (1998).

8 J. Holland *et al.* (1994); C. Roberts, S. Kippax, C. Waldby and J. Crawford, 'Faking it: The Story of 'Ohh!', *Women's Studies International Forum* 18 (5/6) (1995), pp. 523–532.

9 J. Holland *et al.* (1994).

10 D. Tolman (1994). 'Daring to Desire: Culture and the Bodies of Adolescent Girls', in J. Irvine (ed.), *Sexual Cultures and the Construction of Adolescent Identities* (Philadelphia: Temple University Press).

11 R. Thomson and S. Scott (1991).

12 E. Grosz (1994). *Volatile Bodies: Towards a Corporeal Feminism* (Indiana Bloomington: University Press).

13 E. Grosz, 'Notes Towards a Corporeal Feminism', *Australian Feminist Studies: Special Issue, Feminism and the Body* 5 (1987), p. 7.

14 M. Merleau-Ponty (1962). *The Phenomenology of Perception* (trans. Colin Smith) (London: Routledge and Kegan Paul).

15 E. Grosz (1994), p. 87.

16 M. Merleau-Ponty (1962).

17 Subjects are identified by, Method (FG = Focus Group, II = Individual Interview, CA = Couple Activity, Q = Questionnaire), School Status (AS = At School, NAS = Not At School), Age (17 = 17 years, 18 = 18 years, 19 = 19 years).

18 M. Corbett Robinson (1994), p. 70.

19 J. Holland, C. Ramazanoglu and S. Sharpe (1993). 'Wimp or Gladiator: Contradictions in Acquiring Masculine Sexuality', *Women, Risk and AIDS Project, Men Risk and AIDS Project* (London: Tufnell).

20 D. Tolman (1994).

21 S. Williams (1996), p. 23.

22 Ibid., p. 27.

23 Ibid., p. 23.

24 J. Holland *et al.* (1994).

25 Cited in D. Fuss (1989). *Essentially Speaking: Feminism, Nature and Difference* (London: Routledge).

26 J. Holland *et al.* (1994), p. 12.

27 V. Seidler (1997).

28 J. Holland *et al.* (1993), p. 2.

nine

Young Pakeha Men's Conceptions of Health, Illness and Healthcare

1 H. Williams ([1844]1975). *A Dictionary of the Maori Language* (Wellington: A.R. Shearer, Government Printer).

2 National Health Committee (NHC) (1998). *The Social, Cultural and Economic Determinants of Health in New Zealand: Action to Improve Health* (Wellington, The National Advisory Committee on Health and Disability, June).

3 G.J. Armelagos, T. Leatherman, M. Ryan and L. Sibley, 'Biocultural Synthesis in Medical Anthropology', *Medical Anthropology* 14 (1992), pp. 35–52.

4 R. Crawford (1985). 'A Cultural Account of 'Health': Control, Release and the Social Body', in J. McKinley (ed.), *Issues in the Political Economy of Health Care* (New York: Tavistock), pp. 61–103.

5 P. Bourdieu (1984). *Distinction: A Social Critique of the Judgement of Taste* (trans. Richard Nice) (Cambridge, Mass: Harvard University Press); (1990). *Outline of a Theory of Practice* (trans. Richard Nice) (Cambridge: Cambridge University Press); J. Watson (2000). *Male Bodies: Health, Culture, and Identity* (Buckingham and Philadelphia: Open University Press).

6 S. Williams, 'Theorising Class, Health and Lifestyles: Can Bourdieu Help Us?', *Sociology of Health and Illness*, 17 (5) (1995), pp. 577–604.

7 E. Cameron and J. Bernardes (1998). 'Gender and Disadvantage in Health: Mens' Health for a Change', *Sociology of Health and Illness* 20 (5) (1998), pp. 673–693.

8 Ibid.

9 R.W. Connell (1995). *Masculinities* (St. Leonards, NSW: Allen and Unwin).

10 National Health Committee (1998).

11 R.W. Connell (1995); U. Sharma (1997) 'What is an Ethnic Group? The View From Social Anthropolgy', in A. Clarke and E. Parsons (eds), *Culture, Kinship and Genes: Towards Cross-Cultural Genetics* (London: Macmillan Press), p. 78.

12 R. Connell (1983). *Which Way is Up? Essays on Sex, Class and Culture* (Sydney: Allen and Unwin), cited in B. James and K. Saville-Smith (1994). *Gender, Culture and Power: Challenging New Zealand's Gendered Culture* (Auckland: Oxford University Press), p. 52.

13 North Health (1996). *Health Issues for Males in the North Health Region* (Unpublished report, North Health, February).

14 North Health (1996). 'Health issues for males in the North Health Region'. Unpublished report, North Health. February.

15 R. Walker (1998). *People in the North Health Region: A Demographic Profile From the 1996 Census* (Auckland: Health Funding Authority, April).

16 Ministry of Health (1999). *Our Health, Our Future: Hauora Pakari, Koiora Roa: The Health of New Zealanders 1999* (Ministry of Health, Wellington, December).

17 Ibid.

18 J. Park, K. Scott, J. Benseman, and E. Berry (1995). *A Bleeding Nuisance: Living With Haemophilia in Aotearoa New Zealand* (Department of Anthropology, University of Auckland), p. 14.

19 J. Phillips (1996). *A Man's Country: The Image of the Pakeha Male – A History* (Auckland: Penguin).

20 W. Gamble (2000). Portrait of a Captain Who Never Yields. *The New Zealand Herald*, A15. 29th May.

21 Ibid.

22 M. Messner (1992). *Power at Play: Sports and the Problem of Masculinity* (Boston: Beacon Press).

23 J. Park, '"The Worst Hassle is You Can't Play Rugby": Haemophilia and Masculinity in New Zealand', *Current Anthropology*, 41(3) (2000), p. 446.

24 M. Durie, 'A Maori Perspective of Health', *Social Science and Medicine*, 20 (1985), pp. 483–486.

25 Christine Dureau, personal communication.

26 Ministry of Health (1999).

27 A. Parr, R. Whittaker and G. Jackson (1998). *The Northern Region Health Survey 1996/97* (Auckland: Health Funding Authority. June).

28 J. Raeburn and A. Sidaway (1995). *Psychosocial Dimensions of Men's Health: A Review Commissioned by North Health* (Department of Psychiatry and Behavioural Science, University of Auckland).

29 National Health Committee (1998).

30 Youthline (1999). *Consultation with Young People on Sexual and Reproductive Health Issues*. A report for the Ministry of Youth Affairs, Wellington. December.

31 Ibid., p. 56.

32 Ibid., p. 10.

33 Ibid., p. 10.

34 S. Bridgeman (2000). Only Benefits Can Come of Frankness on Prostates. *The New Zealand Herald*, Dialogue, A17. Thursday, 18th May.

35 Ibid.

36 P. Davis and K. Dew. (eds) (1999). *Health and Society in Aotearoa New Zealand*. (Auckland: Oxford).

37 J. Raeburn and A. Sidaway (1995).

38 J. Park (2000), p. 445.

39 G. Ansley (2000). Matt Slade: Broken Ankle. *The New Zealand Herald*, A1, Friday, October 27, p. A1.

40 J. Park (2000).

41 R. Crawford (1985).

42 Ibid.

43 I. Hodges, 'Drinking Vernacular and the Negotiation of Intimacy', *Sites*, 11 (1985), pp. 13–19.

44 R.W. Connell (1995), p. 71.

ten

Abducted By Aliens: Heterosexual Men and Sexual Health

1 While this chapter is indebted to staff at the Auckland Sexual Health Service, Drs Rick Franklin and Murray Reid for their initiative, and Dr Nicky Perkins and Annette Mortensen for their considerable expertise, to co-researcher Reweti Te Mete and reader Ruth Allen, the views represented therein are those of the author and do not purport to represent those of any other researchers or sexual health service staff.

2 See The Institute of Environmental and Scientific Research (ESR) (2000). STD Surveillance Data. Quarterly Reports and Annual Summaries (Wellington: Department of Environmental and Scientific Research).

3 S. Hawkes and G. Hart, 'Men's Sexual Health Matters: Promoting Reproductive Health in an International Context', *Tropical Medicine and International Health*, 5(7) (2000), A37–A44.

4 K. Holmes, P. Mardh, P. Sparling, S. Lemon, W. Stamm, P. Piot and J. Wassrheit (1999). *Sexually Transmitted Diseases*, 3rd ed. (Auckland: McGraw-Hill).

5 Ibid. (1999), p. 109.

6 J. Holland, C. Ramazanolgu, S. Sharpe and R. Thompson (1998). *The Male in the Head: Young People, Heterosexuality and Power* (London: The Tufnell Press).

7 H. Campbell, R. Law and J. Honeyfield (1999). '"What it Means to be a Man": Hegemonic Masculinity and the Reinvention of Beer', in R. Law, H. Campbell and

J. Dolan (eds), *Masculinities in Aotearoa/ New Zealand* (Palmerston North: Dunmore Press).

8 N. Gavey (1991). 'Sexual Victimisation: Prevalence Among New Zealand University Students', *Journal of Consulting and Clinical Psychology* 59 (13) (1991), p. 464ff.

9 A. Wyllie, M. Millard and J.F. Zhang (1996). *Drinking in New Zealand: A National Survey 1995.* (Auckland: Alcohol and Public Health Research Unit, University of Auckland).

10 B. Donovan, 'The Repertoire of Human Efforts to Avoid Sexually Transmissible Diseases – Past and Present: Part 1 Strategies Used Before or Instead of Sex', *Sexually Transmitted Infections*, 76 (2000), pp. 7–12.

11 P. Davis, R. L. Lay-Yee and O. Jacobson (1996). 'Conservatism and Constancy? New Zealand Sexual Culture in the Era of AIDS', in P. Davis (ed.), *Intimate Details and Vital Statistics: AIDS, Sexuality and the Social Order in New Zealand* (Auckland: Auckland University Press), pp. 48–66.

12 J. Baldwin and J. Baldwin, 'Heterosexual Anal Intercourse: An Understudied High Risk Behaviour', *Archives of Sexual Behaviour* 29 (4) (2000), p. 357ff.

13 D. Halperin and R. Bailey, 'Heterosexual Anal Intercourse: Prevalence, Cultural Factors, HIV Infection and Other Health Risks', *AIDS Patient Care STDs* 13 (12) (1999), pp. 717–30.

14 Ministry of Youth Affairs (1998). *Options for Enhancing the Effectiveness of Government Policy on Young People's Sexual and Reproductive Health. An Issues Paper* (Wellington: Ministry of Youth Affairs); (1998b). *Young Men's Involvement in Sexual and Reproductive Health: Current Status and Initiatives* (Wellington: Ministry of Youth Affairs); (2000a). *Increasing Consistent Condom Use By Young Men*. (Wellington: Ministry of Youth Affairs); Ministry of Youth Affairs and Youthline (1999). *Consultation with Young People on Sexual and Reproductive Health Issues For Young Men* (Wellington: Ministry of Youth Affairs).

15 Ministry of Youth Affairs (2000a), p. 18.

16 S. McKernon, 'Managing Condom Use and Non-Use: A Study of Condom Uses Among Clients of a Sexual Health Clinic', *Venereology* 9 (4) (1996), pp. 233–238.

17 Education Review Office (1997). *Reproductive and Sexual Health Education: A Report Provided by the Education Review Office for the Ministry of Health* (Wellington, Education Review Office).

18 K. Elliot (1997). *Adolescent's Perceptions of School Based Sexuality Education Programmes* (Unpublished Masters Thesis. Auckland: University of Auckland).

19 Institute of Environmental and Scientific Research (2000). *STD Surveillance Data. Quarterly Reports and Annual Summaries* (Wellington: Department of Environmental and Scientific Research). Note that this data presents cases reported to ESR only. Data from family planning, student and youth health services is incomplete, and there is no data available from GPs and other community health services including their relevant diagnostic services. Inclusion of this data might change the percentages completely in unpredictable ways. Existing data suggests about 5% of family planning clients and 30% of student and youth health clients are male. Many people present at these latter services for issues other than sexual health specifically.

20 S. Hawkes and G. Hart (2000).

21 Ministry of Health title pages of the following publications: Ministry of Health (1997a). *Sexually Transmitted Diseases, Prevention and Control: the Public Health*

Issues (Wellington, Ministry of Health); (1997b). *Rangatahi Sexual Wellbeing and Reproductive Health: the Public Health Issues* (Wellington, Ministry of Health).

22 P. Davis, R.L. Lay Yee and O. Jacobsen (1996).

23 I. Pool, J. Dickson, A. Dharmalingam, S. Hillcoat-Nalletamby, K. Johnstone and H. Roberts (1999). *New Zealand's Contraceptive Revolutions* (University of Waikato: Population Studies Centre).

24 N. Gavey and K. McPhillips (1999). 'Subject to Romance: Heterosexual Passivity as an Obstacle to Women Initiating Condom Use', *Psychology of Women Quarterly* 23 (2) (1999), pp. 349–367.

25 S. McKernon (1996, 1997).

26 P. Barry *et al.*, 'Partner-Specific Relationship Characteristics and Condom Use Among Young People With Sexually Transmitted Diseases', *The Journal of Sex Research* 37 (1) (2000), pp. 69–75.

27 T. Peterman, L. Lin, D. Newman, M. Kamb, G. Bolan, J. Zenilman, J. Douglas, J. Rogers and C. Malotte, 'Does Measured Behaviour Reflect STD Risk? An Analysis of Data from a Randomised Controlled Behavioural Intervention Study', *Sexually Transmitted Diseases* 27 (8) (2000), pp. 446–451.

28 D. Goetz, 'Durex: Good Sex, Not Just Safe Sex', *Advertising Age* 70 (28) (1999), pp. 12–15.

29 A. Bryan, L. Aiken and S. West (1999). 'The Impact of Males Proposing Condom Use on Perceptions of an Initial Sexual Encounter', *Personality and Social Pyschology Bulletin* 25 (3) (1999), pp. 275–286.

30 S. McKernon and R. Te Mete (2000). *Abducted By Aliens: Men's Experiences Of Auckland Sexual Health Service* (Auckland Sexual Health Service, Auckland Hospital, New Zealand).

31 D. Plummer and B. Forrest, 'Factors Affecting Indigenous Australian's Access to Sexual Health Clinical Services', *Venereology* 12 (2) (1999), pp. 47–51; A. Smith, A. Mischewski and S. Gifford, '"They Just Treat You as a Number": Aspects of Men's Experience in a Melbourne Sexual Health Service', *Venereology* 12 (1) (1999), pp. 16–19.

32 B. Lichtenstein (1996). 'Creating Icons of AIDS: the Media and Popular Culture', in P. Davis (ed.), *Intimate Details and Vital Statistics: AIDS, Sexuality and the Social Order in New Zealand* (Auckland: Auckland University Press); D. Plummer (1999). *Girl's Germs.* Seventh Scientific Chapter Meeting of the Australasian College of Sexual Health Physicians, Sydney, Australia.

33 A.C. Mortensen (2000). *Destigmatisation: A Grounded Theory of the Practice of Sexual Health Nurses*. A thesis submitted for the degree of Master of Philosophy in Nursing, Massey University.

34 Hook, *et al.*, 'Delayed Presentation to Clinics for Sexually Transmitted Diseases by Symptomatic Patients: a Potential Contributor to Continuing STD Morbidity', *Sexually Transmitted Diseases* 24 (8) (September) (1997), pp. 443–8.

35 R.W. Connell (1998). *Maculinities* (Berkeley: University of California Press).

Index